Diarrhoeal Disease and Malnutrition:
A Clinical Update

Diarrhoeal Disease and Malnutrition:
A CLINICAL UPDATE

EDITED BY

Michael Gracey MD (Syd), PhD (W.Aust), FRACP
Associate Professor of Child Health, University of Western Australia;
Director, Gastroenterology and Nutrition Research Unit,
Princess Margaret Children's Medical Research Foundation,
Perth, Western Australia

FOREWORD BY

Charlotte M. Anderson MD, MSc, FRACP, FRCP
Emeritus Professor of Paediatrics and Child Health, University of Birmingham;
Honorary Research Fellow, Department of Child Health,
University of Western Australia

CHURCHILL LIVINGSTONE
EDINBURGH LONDON MELBOURNE AND NEW YORK 1985

CHURCHILL LIVINGSTONE
Medical Division of Longman Group Limited

Distributed in the United States of America by
Churchill Livingstone Inc., 1560 Broadway, New York,
N.Y. 10036, and by associated companies, branches and
representatives throughout the world.

First published 1985

ISBN 0 443 02892 3

British Library Cataloguing in Publication Data
Diarrhoeal disease and malnutrition : a
    clinical update.
    1. Diarrhea in children
    I. Gracey, Michael
    618.92'3427   RJ456.D5

Library of Congress Cataloging in Publication Data
Main entry under title:
Diarrhoeal disease and malnutrition.
    Includes index.
    1. Diarrhea in children. 2. Intestines — Infections.
3. Malnutrition in children — Developing countries.
I. Gracey, Michael.   [DNLM: 1. Diarrhea — in infancy &
childhood. 2. Nutrition Disorders — in infancy &
childhood.   WS 312 D5393]
RJ456.D5D53   1985   618.92'3427   84-21412

Produced by Longman Singapore Publishers (Pte) Ltd.
Printed in Singapore.

Foreword

It gives me considerable pleasure to write a foreword for such a timely volume as this clinical update edited by Michael Gracey. I am proud to have had some initial influence on his interest and work in diarrhoeal disease of children.

During the last several decades a transformation has taken place in our understanding of acute diarrhoea. Some 40 years ago, as a junior house physician at the Royal Children's Hospital, Melbourne, one of my busiest and most demanding posts was the care of patients with diarrhoea. Gastroenteritis was still a common condition then, even in a developed community, especially in the summer. The number of patients with diarrhoea was also boosted at that time by child refugees from war-ravaged Europe in whom malnutrition was a complicating factor. We were still taught that rest for the bowel was indicated, so deprivation of oral feedings until diarrhoea ceased was common practice; fluids were administered intravenously but the precise electrolyte composition of the fluid was still a matter for discussion. Oral fluids were not resumed until diarrhoea had ceased for 24–48 hours and then followed a slow re-grading on to oral feeds from sugar and water to the infant's normal strength feedings, usually involving a hospital stay of 10–14 days with considerable deprivation of calories during that time. Known infecting agents were confined to salmonella and shigella as cholera was not a problem in our setting. Viruses were suspected but not identified.

During the intervening years, many more infective agents have been recognised and their method of inducing diarrhoea has been clarified through a progressive understanding of the normal mechanisms involved in fluid and electrolyte absorption and secretion in the intestine. This has resulted in a complete change in attitude to initial management, in that replacement of fluid losses by the oral route is commenced at the onset of the condition and patients are not deprived of oral intake until diarrhoea ceases. Recognition of the relationship of undernutrition to impairment of intestinal immune mechanisms as one of the factors involved in the high recurrence rate of diarrhoeal episodes in young children in the developing world has been of considerable importance.

In the western world, gastroenteritis wards in children's hospitals are now small and often underpopulated; mortality from gastroenteritis is minor compared to that from birth defects and accidents. However, this is still far from the situation in the developing world as the chapters of Dr Mata of Costa Rica and Dr Merson of the World Health Organization indicate in this volume. The horrifying extent of mortality, morbidity and health care expenditure caused by childhood diarrhoea in these countries is still a major cause of concern and the rationale for the WHO Programme of Control of Diarrhoeal Diseases.

In the early 1950s I was a research fellow at the Birmingham Children's Hospital in England when Dr Keith Rogers first recorded epidemics in young infants of acute diarrhoea related to coliform organisms which were previously considered to be inhabitants of the normal gut. These, however, were particular strains of *E. coli* known as 'enteropathogenic' and designated by various serotyping numbers. His painstaking and careful recording of the spread through the infant wards of one of these organisms, was a fine lesson in epidemiology. At that stage we still had no real understanding of why such organisms could produce profuse fluid loss in the stools but 'colonic hurry' from irritation of the bowel wall was assumed. The important work of Thomson in the 1940s, showing that these enteropathogenic *E. coli* multiplied in the normally sterile upper small intestine had little impact on medical workers and it was left to the veterinary scientists to recognise that some of these so-called enteropathogenic organisms produced toxins which had an effect on fluid movement across the mucosa of the small intestine. Study of the mode of action of the toxins was stimulated by veterinarians' interest in acute diarrhoeal illnesses which caused considerable mortality in piglets and very young calves.

Considerable and rapid increase in our understanding of enzymatic transport and immune processes of the small intestinal mucosa, aided by many new biochemical and technological procedures, one of which was the introduction of peroral intestinal mucosal biopsy in the late 1950s, has yielded much valuable information in human studies. At first this knowledge obtained by workers in western countries was applied to the study of chronic diarrhoeal and malabsorptive states among their own populations, an example of this being the recognition of the relationship of certain dietary sugars to persistent fluid diarrhoea. The rare inborn errors of development of disaccharidase enzymes, such as sucrase and lactase, were first to be described. Very soon afterwards it was realised that disaccharidase deficiency, particularly of lactase, was important in prolonging the diarrhoea which occurs in some infants following acute gastroenteritis. Workers in developing countries were quick to follow up these findings in their own populations and in so doing were also instrumental in clarifying the differences in behaviour of the enzyme lactase in communities of differing racial origins, discussed in the chapter by Professor Ransome-Kuti.

In the late 1960s and early 70s, western research workers were becoming increasingly interested in studying diarrhoeal diseases in the developing world and at the same time young medical and scientific graduates from these developing countries sought training in gastroenterological diseases of children. A very welcome co-operation between the two groups of workers was built up, aided considerably by such bodies as WHO, the British Council, the Rockefeller Foundation and other American and European institutions.

The most important observation of this period came from the then Cholera Research Laboratory in Dhaka, Bangladesh, where it was first shown that fluid losses from choleraic diarrhoea could be successfully offset by oral rehydration therapy (ORT) with glucose or sucrose and electrolyte mixtures commenced at the onset of diarrhoea and vigorously pursued during the illness. Co-operation with American workers rapidly led to demonstration of the mechanism by which cholera toxin stimulated secretion of fluid and electrolyte from the epithelial cells of the small intestine whilst leaving unharmed the transport of sodium coupled glucose and water. This has been described as potentially the most important medical advance this century. Understanding of the effect of toxins of other organisms such as the coliforms quickly followed.

In the early 1970s came the documentation of viruses as causes of acute diarrhoea, notably the rotavirus. The demonstration of rotavirus particles in small intestinal epithelial cells and in the stools were examples of the application of technological advance — in this case the electron microscope — to material already being studied by workers independently and respectively in Melbourne and Birmingham.

Following the success of oral rehydration therapy for choleraic diarrhoea, workers in developing countries were quick to apply this technique to diarrhoeal diseases caused by other agents with marked success. Gut rest was finally laid to rest but it has taken considerably longer for western medical personnel to accept that ORT could be applied (with some exceptions) to diarrhoeal states in their own populations.

In May 1978 WHO, when announcing its commitment to primary health care and to the World Health Assembly call for Health for All by the Year 2000, launched a Diarrhoeal Diseases Control Programme aimed at co-ordinating all this new knowledge with the object, in the short term, of reducing mortality from such conditions in young children in the developing world and in the longer term preventing malnutrition and improving environmental hygiene and the delivery of health care amongst such populations.

Michael Gracey, the editor of this update, is an admirable example of a western trained paediatric gastroenterologist who has used his knowledge and technical skills to help in combating the major problem of diarrhoeal disease and undernutrition amongst the scattered urban and rural Aboriginal population of the vast State of Western Australia and in neighbouring countires in South East Asia. As regards this volume he is to be congratulated, firstly, on bringing together data, often only available in diverse medical journals and conference proceedings and, secondly, on choosing such an excellent group of contributors who have been able to present their data in such a readable fashion. This book is highly suitable for practising paediatricians and physicians and also a wide range of other health workers. There are excellent chapters covering the aspects referred to in this foreword, as well as the detailed practical application of ORT, a critical assessment of other means of controlling diarrhoeal fluid loss, long-term prospects for control and prevention by widespread immunisation measures as well as measures necessary to improve the environmental and nutritional background in which diarrhoeal disease flourishes in children in developing countries. Control of diarrhoea by medical means must be accompanied by control of hygiene in the environment, production and distribution of food and delivery of health care to all, otherwise medical knowledge will still not be properly utilised.

This book is truly an update in our current knowledge of diarrhoeal diseases and I hope it becomes widely used in both developed and developing medical centres and by workers in the field.

Perth, Western Australia   Charlotte M. Anderson
1985

Preface

One of mankind's major scourages, smallpox, has recently been eradicated. Others, including diphtheria and whooping cough, respond well to immunization strategies; other diseases, such as tuberculosis and staphylococcal infections can now be treated successfully with specific antimicrobial therapy. However, for millions of the world's children, the dual and sinister synergistic insults of diarrhoeal disease and malnutrition still persist and exact an horrific toll annually. These unpleasant bedfellows are the subject of this book.

In the past ten years such a lot has been written about diarrhoeal diseases and malnutrition that it has become almost impossible for the non-specialist reader to keep up with the literature. The main aim of this book is to bring the interested reader up to date with important advances which have occurred in that decade in these related fields, particularly about acute childhood diarrhoea. It is, thus, designed as a real *clinical update* for paediatricians, other doctors, nurses, primary health workers, public health workers, medical administrators and policy makers to be made aware of the most important recent advances and selected sources for further reading. The topics covered include epidemiology, mechanisms causing diarrhoea, 'newer' pathogenic organisms, immunization, oral rehydration therapy, public health programmes and the World Health Organization's approach to control of diarrhoeal diseases, world-wide.

Throughout the book we try to focus on diarrhoeal diseases as a serious and prevalent clinical problem in areas where childhood malnutrition is still widespread. This is not a textbook about childhood malnutrition or about childhood gastroenteritis. It is, rather, a discussion of the major areas where our knowledge about these synergistic conditions has improved over recent years and where we can realistically expect future improvements, of practical importance, to occur over the forseeable future.

I am exceptionally fortunate, as editor of this small volume, to have had the support of prominent and very busy colleagues in scattered parts of the world and in diverse professional fields, to realise the publisher's aim of adopting a multi-disciplinary approach to a very complex and sensitive medico-social problem. I thank my co-authors most sincerely for their help but, as editor, I must accept overall responsibility for this book's shortcomings.

This book is dedicated to the children of the world's poor.

Perth, Western Australia   Michael Gracey
1985

Contributors

Helen M. Berschneider DVM

Division of Digestive Diseases and Nutrition, School of Medicine, University of North Carolina, Chapel Hill, USA

Deborah Blum BA, MD, MSc

Lecturer, London School of Hygiene & Tropical Medicine, London

William A.M. Cutting FRCP (Ed), DCH RCPS (Glas), DObst RCOG

Senior Lecturer in Tropical Child Health, Edinburgh University

Michael Gracey MD(Syd), PhD(W Aust), FRACP

Associate Professor Child Health, University of Western Australia, and Director, Gastroenterology and Nutrition Research Unit, Princess Margaret Children's Medical Research Foundation, Perth, Western Australia

David I. Grove MD, FRACP, DTM&H

Associate Professor of Medicine, University of Western Australia, Perth, Western Australia

Sai Kit Lam PhD

Associate Professor; Director, WHO Collaborating Centre for Reference and Research (Dengue and DHF), Department of Medical Microbiology. University of Malaya, Kuala Lumpur 22–11, Malaysia

Myron M. Levine MD, DTPH

Professor of Medicine and Pediatrics. Director, Center for Vaccine Development, University of Maryland School of Medicine

Charles R. Madeley MD, MRCPath

Professor of Clinical Virology, University of Newcastle; Consultant Virologist, Newcastle Health Authority

Dilip Mahalanabis MB, BS, FRCPE

Diarrhoeal Diseases Control Programme, World Health Organization, Switzerland

Leonardo Mata DSc

Director, Instituto de Investigaciones en Salud (INISA), Universidad De Costa Rica

Michael H. Merson MD

Director, Diarrhoeal Diseases Control Programme, World Health Organization

D. W. Powell MD

Professor of Medicine and Chief, Division of Digestive Diseases & Nutrition, School of Medicine, University of North Carolina, Chapel Hill, USA

Olikoye Ransome-Kuti MB, FRCP(Ed), FMCPaed(Nigeria)

Professor of Paediatrics and Primary Care, Director, Institute of Child Health and Primary Care, College of Medicine, University of Lagos, Nigeria

Michael G. M. Rowland MB, BS, DCH, DTM&H, FRCP

Senior Scientist, Medical Research Council, UK

Robert M. Suskind MD

Professor and Chairman, Department of Pediatrics, College of Medicine, University of South Alabama, Mobile, Alabama, USA

John N. Udall MD, PhD

Assistant Professor, Department of Pediatrics, Harvard Medical School, Boston, Massachusetts, USA

Contents

Global importance of diarrhoeal diseases and malnutration

INTRODUCTION

The amount of new knowledge accumulated in the past 15 years about the aetiology, epidemiology, and public significance of diarrhoeal disease is quite remarkable, particularly because such knowledge has challenged orthodox concepts strongly rooted in misconceptions. Until recently, most diarrhoeas in the general population were regarded as 'food indigestion' and accordingly were given a variety of lay names. Remarkably, even today some medical professionals may refer to certain diarrhoeas as caused by unwholesome food with characteristics incompatible with health. Even though shigellosis, salmonellosis, cholera, giardiasis, amoebiasis, and other specific clinical entities had been characterized satisfactorily, as recently as 10 years ago it was difficult to prove that most outbreaks of diarrhoea in communities were of an infectious origin. In fact, some spoke of 'nutritional diarrhoea' in analogy with nutritional anaemias. It is now accepted, however, that most diarrhoeas in the community and in outpatient and emergency hospital services are related to viral, microbial, and parasitic agents, a concept supported by the following considerations: (a) diarrhoeas are prevalent in ecosystems with inadequate environmental sanitation, education, income, and personal hygiene; (b) secondary cases develop in contacts of index cases within intervals compatible with incubation periods, pointing to spread by direct or indirect contact; (c) incidence and severity of diarrhoea decrease with age, and older persons are relatively free of diarrhoea, suggesting the development of immunity; (d) comprehensive laboratory investigations demonstrate a potential infectious pathogen in about 70 per cent of acute diarrhoea cases (Mata 1983a). Thus, improvement of personal hygiene and environmental sanitation results in a significant reduction in morbidity and mortality due to diarrhoeal diseases. It is easy to understand the epidemic proportions of diarrhoea in New York City at the turn of the century, comparable to that of many less developed countries today, when environmental conditions, education, personal hygiene, and income were low, especially among immigrants.

Part of the gap regarding the aetiology of diarrhoea was resolved in the

1

last 20 years with the discovery of new agents such as rotaviruses, non-cultivatable adenoviruses, 27 nm agents, caliciviruses, coronaviruses, and enterotoxigenic Enterobacteriaceae (see Mata 1983a). Concomitantly, already known agents were rediscovered in diarrhoea cases, namely, *Campylobacter jejuni, Cryptosporidium muris*, and *Yersinia enterocolitica* (WHO 1980). Furthermore, plasmids with the capacity to induce virulence in *Aeromonas hydrophila, Klebsiella*, and other Enterobacteriaceae were characterized, while 140 MD plasmid-carrying bacteria were shown to invade the intestinal mucosa causing a dysenteric syndrome.

Proliferation of bacteria in the upper small intestine of man in tropical and subtropical areas is associated with chronic diarrhoea and malabsorption especially in severely malnourished children (Gracey 1979). However, bacterial overgrowth of the small intestine is a common finding in apparently normal individuals in less developed countries. Peace Corps volunteers who suffer from diarrhoea, malabsorption and weight loss, also exhibit bacterial proliferation which disappears upon resettlement in an urban sanitary environment (Lindebaum et al 1971). Finally, it is probable that some *Mycoplasma, Chlamydia* and other viruses (and viroids?) are involved in the aetiology of diarrhoea.

INTERACTION BETWEEN DIARRHOEAL DISEASES AND MALNUTRITION

The frequent pathogenic infections and the bacterial overgrowth of the small intestine of humans living in poverty reflect the close relationship between the quality of food consumed, the nutritional status and diarrhoea. Probably most diarrhoeas in less developed countries are acquired by ingesting contaminated foods and water. Person-to-person spread by hands, and indirect transmission via utensils, flies, and fomites, also play a role (Table 1.1). Environmental and cultural factors favoring transmission of diarrheal diseases, simultaneously deprive the host of an adequate diet and of the physical and social stimulation required for optimal food utilization.

The interrelation between diarrhoea and malnutrition was not clear until recently, partly because the universal concern with food scarcity led to the belief, without sound evidence, that malnutrition is due to inadequate food consumption alone, without consideration of other environmenatal determinants. When Scrimshaw et al (1959) published their pioneering work on

Table 1.1 Transmission of diarrhoeal disease agents

Anus (faeces) — fingers — mouth
Anus (faeces) — fingers (foods, drinking water, utensils) — mouth
Anus (faeces) — aerosols (fingers, foods, drinking water, utensils, objects) — mouth
Anus (faeces) — fomites (fingers, foods, drinking water) — mouth
Anus (faeces) — soil (water, foods, drinking water, utensils) — mouth
Anus (faeces) — soil (insects, foods, drinking water, utensils) — mouth
Anus — mouth

nutrition-infection interactions, some attention was turned to infectious diseases in the aetiology of malnutrition. The role of infection in the genesis of chronic and severe malnutrition is now recognized by most experienced pediatricians, as had been recognized by Cicely Williams in her classical description of kwashiorkor in the 1930s. Long-term prospective observation of children in their rural ecosytems has now revealed the importance of infectious diseases, particularly diarrhoea, in the development of chronic malnutrition and its acute forms, and in the occurrence of premature death of infants and young children (Mata 1978, Black et al 1982a).

One must consider the intestine as a collection of microbial habitats inhabited by myriads of protozoa, yeasts and bacteria, and also susceptible to being invaded by dozens of helminths, pathogenic bacteria and viruses. The various microbial habitats include the lumen and interplical spaces; plicae and villi which are much more numerous in the duodenum, jejunum, and proximal ileum than in the terminal ileum and colon; intervillous spaces offering opportunities for microbial attachment and for cell invasion; and millions of delicate villi lined by goblet cells, extruding cells and nutrients. In malnutrition, chronic malabsorption and other pathologic processes, there is formation of hollow spaces or microcaverns, possibly permitting stagnation of secretions and cell debris. Bacteria and protozoa associate with crypt cells and dwell in the crypt, or adhere to the villous epithelium, usually at the tips. Agents may be loosely or strongly associated with the host mucosa. *Cryptosporidium* attaches to the brush border of enterocytes, dwelling under the microcalyx. *Giardia* firmly adheres to the mucosal surface and causes anatomical and functional alterations associated with malabsorption. Other agents invade epithelial cells and burrow into the lamina propria, where they cause an inflammatory response with abscess formation and eventual mucosal ulceration. Finally, other micro-organisms translocate to reach the lymph and blood circulation, homing in on distant organs, as in salmonellosis (see Mata 1983b).

It is easy, then, to accept that the close host-parasite interactions will be translated into important physiological and nutritional abnormalities. The negative nutritional effects of diarrhoea are reduced food consumption, reduced nutrient absorption, increased secretion, protein-losing enteropathy, metabolic alterations, growth retardation, and severe energy-protein malnutrition (Table 1.2) (Mata et al 1980).

Reduced food consumption

Diarrhoea interferes with proper consumption of the usual diet, an effect due to one or more of the following symptoms and signs: anorexia, vomiting, dehydration, fever, discomfort, and anxiety. Furthermore, cultural traditions and beliefs often result in parental suppression of foods for days or weeks after an attack of diarrhoea. Prospective observations in cohorts of Guatemalan and Costa Rican rural children living under contrasting en-

Table 1.2 Effect of diarrhoeal disease on the host nutrition, growth and development, and health and survival

Nutrition
Reduced food consumption
Impaired digestion
Impaired absorption
Increased secretion
Metabolic alterations

Growth and development
Acute weight loss
Arrest of linear (height) growth
Progressive wasting and stunting
Impaired interaction with attendants
Impaired learning

Health and survival
Precipitation of severe malnutrition
Impaired immune function
Increased hospitalization, disability and absenteeism
Decreased survival

Table 1.3 Clinical features associated with reduced food consumption, children with diarrhoea observed from birth to 2 years (Puriscal, Costa Rica, 1979–1981)

Diarrhoea	No. of episodes	Number (%) with			
		Anorexia	Fever	Vomiting	Dehydration
Rotavirus	43	15(35)	22(51)	18(42)	4(9)
Campylobacter	17	8(47)	7(41)	6(35)	0
Shigella	6	3(50)	3(50)	0	0
Total	66	26(39)	32(48)	24(36)	4(6)

vironmental conditions revealed that anorexia and vomiting commonly accompany diarrhoea (Table 1.3) often causing severe restriction of food intake for days or weeks (Mata et al 1980). Weekly dietary surveys in weaned children showed that as much as 20 to 50 per cent of the available home diet is not consumed when diarrhoea strikes (Table 1.4) (Mata 1979, Whitehead 1981). Bengali workers demonstrated that the effect had diminished two weeks after recuperation, but was not corrected then, specially in rotavirus and enterotoxigenic *Escherichia coli* (ETEC) diarrhoea (Molla

Table 1.4 Mean daily food consumption during acute diarrhoeal disease in Guatemalan and Ugandan children

Age (months)	Guatemala*				Uganda+	
	Protein (g)		Energy (MJ)		Energy (MJ)	
	Well	*Diarrhoea*	*Well*	*Diarrhoea*	*Well*	*Diarrhoea*
25–30	25	19	3.82	3.02	3.52	1.89
31–36					3.95	2.03
% Change well-diarrhoea		24		21		48

* After Mata (1979)
+After Whitehead (1981)

et al 1983a). This observation is particularly relevant to developing countries, because children who are chronically malnourished frequently consume quantities of food that are just adequate for normal growth.

Reduced absorption of nutrients

Diarrhoea impairs consumption and absorption of macronutrients, an effect persisting for several weeks after the episode. Adhesion of bacteria to the mucosa, release of enterotoxins, direct damage to the enterocyte and crypt cells, bacterial hydrolysis of bile acids and carbohydrates, and other pathogenic actions result in a diminished capacity of the mucosa to absorb macro- and micronutrients. Molla and coworkers (1983b) recently showed a decreased absorption of nitrogen, calories, fat, and carbohydrate in children with specific diarrhoeas, an effect partially corrected eight weeks after termination of the episode.

Increased secretion

Diarrhoea is also a state of hypersecretion. In rotavirus infection there is a clear movement of water from the infected segment of the small intestine into the lumen, resulting in a decreased sodium flux from the lumen to the extracellular fuid (e.c.f.) and an increased sodium flux from the e.c.f. into the lumen (Field 1976). These alterations are related to damage and lysis of villous tips with replacement of absorptive enterocytes by immature crypt cells. There is no alteration of cyclic adenosine monophosphate (CMP) concentrations. Other causes of hypersecretion are stimulation of cyclic AMP and cyclic guanosine monophosphate (GMP) by heat-labile toxins and heat-stable toxins released by enteric bacteria, or by increased bile and fatty acids from bacterial metabolism, or by hormones and neurotransmitters (Table 1.2). The hypersecretory state results in important deficits in sodium, potassium, chloride, and water, and probably in other elements such as vitamins and trace elements.

Nutrient losses

Similar to the abrupt fall in plasma albumin observed after an attack of measles, a 'protein-losing enteropathy' occurs after structural alterations in the mucosal epithelium caused by *shigella*, rotaviruses, and probably *campylobacter, yersinia* and *cryptosporidium*. An increased ratio of α_1-antitrypsin (stool over serum concentrations) was observed in about half of rotavirus diarrhoeas and even more frequently in shigellosis (Rahaman & Wahed 1983). The consequences for malnourished children might be more serious, because in chronic malnutrition there is already a marked thinning of the intestinal wall. The protein-losing enteropathy might help to explain the outbreaks of kwashiorkor that follow by a few weeks the epidemics of diarrhoea. Other metabolic alterations, such as those described in systemic infections, are expected: negative balances of nitrogen, magnesium, potassium, and phosphorus; mobilization of amino acids from muscle for gluconeogenesis; augmented synthesis of acute-phase reactant proteins; and sequestration of trace elements.

Effect on growth and development

Diarrhoea induces acute weight loss and arrest in linear growth, as do other infections. Detailed observation of this phenomenon was possible by prospective studies of children in their natural village ecosystems in Guatemala, the Gambia, Uganda, Bangladesh and Costa Rica (Mata 1978, Martorell et al 1980, Cole & Parkin 1977, Black et al 1982a, Mata 1982). Inspection of individual growth curves of 45 cohort children showed a consistent pattern of relative absence of diarrhoea during exclusive breastfeeding; the nutritional status of infants was adequate, even in those that had experienced fetal growth retardation or were born prematurely (Mata, 1979; Mata, 1982). With the onset of weaning (a protracted process starting at about 3 to 6 months of life and continuing throughout the second year of life) a variety of infections associated with faltering of the weight and height curves were recorded in each child (Mata 1978). Previous description of 20 growth histories selected among the 45 cohort children revealed a consistent pattern of progressive weight deterioration (wastage) with infections. Figure 1.1 depicts the weight curve (compared to the Boston-Iowa 50th percentile), intestinal infections, illnesses and growth increments of a typical Guatemalan village child during his first 3 years of life (Mata et al 1971). This particular boy grew well during the first 6 to 7 months of life, a period characterized by intensive and almost exclusive breast-feeding, and by uncommon and transient enteric infections. *Giardia* appeared at about 6 months of age, but enteroviruses were isolated from early life. Weaning in this particular child peaked at 18 months, and this was accompanied by frequent infections with a variety of enteric agents. This child had in the first 3 years of life: 4 weeks with adenoviruses, 84 with enteroviruses, 8 with *Shigella*, 1 with enteropathogenic *Escherichia coli*, 18 with *Entamoeba histolytica*, 12 with *Giardia*, and 52 with *Ascaris*. He also had 5 weeks with rotaviruses (Mata et al 1983). The child suffered from a continuum of diarrhoeal and respiratory diseases. Weight faltered after six months of age and did not improve during the whole weaning period (6 to 18 months). Thereafter a relative catch-up was observed, but at the end of the third year of life, weight losses were recorded in conjunction with diarrhoea and bronchopneumonia. The child survived the hazards of early childhood, but died of typhoid fever during school years. Similar children succumbed in early childhood (Mata 1978).

The wasting and stunting effect of diarrhoea was more marked in children who had experienced fetal growth retardation, a common event in Guatemalan Indian villages (Mata et al 1980). A negative effect of diarrhoea on

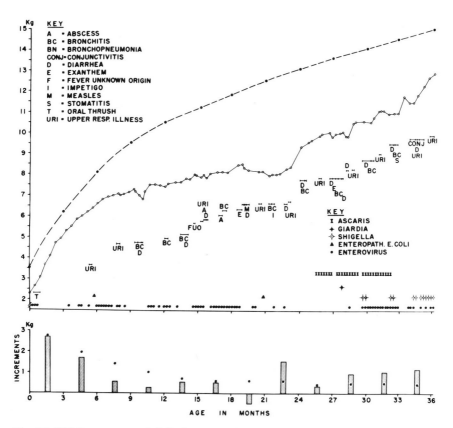

Fig. 1.1 Weight curve, enteric infections and infectious diseases in male child no. 12 of the Cauqué study. *Top*: Broken line is the 50th percentile of the Boston-Iowa growth standard; continuous line is the weight curve of the child. Horizontal bars indicate episodes of disease, and length of bars their duration .Each mark shows a week positive for a particular infectious agent. Note that acute diarrhoeal and acute respiratory infections often occur simultaneously or in succession. *Bottom*: Observed trimester weight increments in the child (vertical bars) and expected median increments of the standard curve (dots). (After Mata et al 1971.)

growth has been described in several other studies. On the other hand, wasted and/or stunted children are prone to suffer from a more severe course of diarrhoea and also exhibit a higher risk of death, as evidenced in field studies in Guatemala, India, Bangladesh and The Gambia (Table 1.5) (Chen et al 1980). Thus, diarrhoea is a malnourishing event, and malnutrition in turn enhances the risk of dying from infection, a costly vicious circle.

THE GLOBAL PROBLEM OF DIARRHOEA

Morbidity estimates

Few studies to measure diarrhoeal diseases morbidity have been conducted. Furthermore, the few available studies used different field methodologies

Table 1.5   Mortality rate according to nutritional status, preschool children, Bangladesh, 1975–1976

Nutritional status as % of Harvard values	Number of children	Deaths per 1000 children 0–11*	12–23*
Weight/height			
>90	399	35.1	17.5
80–89	979	26.6	26.6
70–79	566	28.3	21.2
<70	75	66.7	80.0
Height/age			
>95	182	16.5	16.5
90–94	656	22.9	16.8
85–89	713	28.0	9.8
<85	468	51.3	62.0

*Months after anthropometric assessment
Adapted from Chen et al (1980)

and do not necessarily reflect the world-wide situation. The prospective field study in a small Mayan village in Guatemala concluded that children suffer about eight episodes of diarrhoea per child per year during the first three years of life (Mata et al 1978). A similar figure has been recorded for children also studied prospectively in Matlab, Bangladesh (Black et al 1982a). More recently, even higher rates than those of Cauqué and Matlab were found in Brazilian children by Dr Richard Guerrant (personal communication).

Rohde & Northrup (1976) estimated for 1975, 500 million cases of diarrhoea for children less than 5 years in Africa, Asia and Latin America, an estimate that could well reflect only acute and severe attacks. Another conservative estimate based on 3 studies that employed bi-monthly home visits for surveillance yielded 460 million cases of diarrhoea for 1975, roughly about 1 episode per child per year. However, using the Cauqué data obtained through weekly surveillance, the resulting figure is about 2 billion cases per year (Mata et al 1980). A more recent estimate of the global morbidity based on 5 studies yielded, for 1980, about 1000 million episodes for children under 5 years of age (Snyder & Merson 1982).

Mortality estimates

An investigation into the causes of death in 4 Guatemalan rural communities in 1956–1957, revealed that 43 per cent of the diarrhoeal deaths were not recorded at all in the official vital statistics (Béhar et al 1958). Thus, figures for diarrhoeal disease deaths probably are understimated in less developed countries, although registration of the event and cause has steadily improved over recent years in most nations.

Global estimates of diarrhoeal disease mortality have ranged from 5 to 18 million deaths for children under 5 years of age in 1975 for Africa, Asia and Latin America (Rhode & Northrup 1976). Different ways to estimate the diarrhoea death toll coincided in establishing about 5 million deaths per year, which correspond to about 30 per cent of all deaths in the 0–5 year age group (Puffer & Serrano 1973, Barua 1981, Snyder & Merson 1982).

There is even less information on the relative contribution of the specific diarrhoeas to global morbidity and mortality, and not one single study can be considered representative of the urban and rural situation of any country. The aetiology of diarrhoea varies according to urban or rural setting, season, and level of environmental sanitation and personal hygiene. When these factors are deficient, shigellosis and enterotoxigenic diarrhoeas become very common and are dangerous (Black et al 1982b, Mata et al 1983). The toxic shigellosis and dehydrating bacterial and rotaviral diarrhoeas are likely to account for most deaths in the poor urban settings. The severity and outcome of all diarrhoeas is aggravated by low birth weight, premature weaning, child neglect and other social aberrations that seem to occur more frequently in urban than in rural settings.

Mortality in the Americas

The data of diarrhoeal disease mortality for Latin America appears to be fairly complete (OPS 1980, WHO 1982) as compared to those for Africa. Marked differences are noted between the very low rate in North America and in the rest of the continent (Table 1.6). The highest rate corresponds to Middle America (Mexico and the six Republics of the Isthmus) and tropical South America (which excludes Argentina, Chile, Uruguay and Paraguay). However, even in the Caribbean and in temperate South America, diarrhoea deaths account for a significant part of the total mortality among infants and young children. Thus, diarrhoeal diseases still are a leading cause of death in the Americas (Table 1.7) including the United States and Canada where they ranked 5th as recently as 1976 (OPS 1980, WHO 1982).

Table 1.6 Diarrhoeal disease mortality in the Americas (per 100 000) and proportionate mortality (%), by age, 1976

Region	Age (years) <1 Rate	%	1–4 Rate	%
North (without Mexico)	19	1.4	0.6	0.9
Caribbean	439	15.2	28	15.0
Middle America	1078	22.8	154	25.8
South, tropical	1066	20.3	151	21.5
South, temperate	496	10.9	20	9.1

Adapted from Organización Panamericana de la Salud 1980

Table 1.7   Rank of diarrhoeal disease as a cause of death in the Americas, 1976

Region	Number of nations	Cause of death				
		1st	2nd	3rd	4th	5th
North (without Mexico)	2					1
Caribbean	7		4		3	
Middle America	7	3	2	2		
South, tropical	5	2	3			
South, temperate	3		1	1	1	

Adapted from Organización Panamericana de la Salud 1980

THE GLOBAL PROBLEM OF MALNUTRITION

There is no quantitative information about the contribution of diarrhoeal disease to the genesis of chronic and severe malnutrition, although there is adequate evidence attesting to its contributory role. Cross-cultural studies of mortality and long-term prospective observations have shown the frequent association of diarrhoea and malnutrition in the event of death. The Pan American Study of Childhool Mortality reveled that low birth weight, premature weaning, and postnatal malnutrition were correlates in most diarrhoeal deaths (Puffer & Serrano 1973).

During 8 years of prospective observations on all infants and preschool children in a typical Guatemalan village, 58 child deaths (excluding neonatal) were recorded of which 11 (19 per cent) were diarrhoea-associated and 4 (7 percent) were malnutrition-associated; 3 of the deaths were attributed to both diarrhoea and malnutrition (Mata 1978). In this study, the proficiency of the peadiatrician (Dr J. J. Urrutia) and his field staff probably prevented many deaths from malnutrition and diarrhoea.

It is logical, then, to accept that diarrhoeal disease is a significant contributor to the global rates of malnutrition. The world prevalence of malnutrition compiled by the Nutrition Unit of the World Health Organization is shown in Table 1.8. There seems to be no doubt that a significant proportion of childhood malnutrition is directly or indirectly due to the high rates of diarrhoeal disease prevalent in in the same regions where malnutrition exists. Protein-energy malnutrition is exposed or aggravated in certain regions and countries by food shortages. Nevertheless, since most of the wasting and stunting observed in less developed countries is confined to infants and preschool children, who also are the most severely affected by diarrhoeal and other infectious diseases, a strong causal relationship between infection and malnutrition is sought (Mata 1982).

Iron-deficiency anaemias also are complicated by infections, and in many cases are caused entirely by them (e.g. hookworm infection). Regarding low birth weight, the stunting of child-bearing women frequently is the result of chronic malnutrition and this, in turn, may be induced by repetetive infections during childhood. Therefore, early infectious experiences in child-

Table 1.8 Prevalence of nutritional deficiencies in the developing world

	Africa	Asia[+]	The Americas[§]
Low birth weight	15[*]	27	11
	(3)	(13)	(1)
Weight deficit, preschool children	30	47[‡]	28
	(20)	(94)	(13)
Stunting, preschool children	35	40[‡]	43
	(24)	(81)	(20)
Iron-deficiency anemia, women	40	58	17
	(37)	(172)	(13)

[*] Percentage; in parentheses, millions of persons
[+] Excluding China
[‡] Weighted for India
[§] Excluding Argentina, Chile, Uruguay and Paraguay
Adapted from WHO A36/7 (1983)

hood must have a late indirect repercussion during reproductive age by favouring low birth weight.

Infectious diarrhoea has been recognized as a precipitating factor of severe malnutrition, especially the oedematous form; severe eye manifestations of vitamin A deficiency often appear following diarrhoea and other infectious diseases like measles.

CONTROL OF DIARRHOEAL DISEASES AND MALNUTRITION

There is no doubt that the control and prevention of diarrhoeal diseases will rapidly lead to improved levels of child nutrition and survival. The comparison of diarrhoeal disease death rates throughout the world provides a clue to the marked reduction in mortality in several countries in recent times. Data for the Americas for the period 1967–1977 permit estimation of the change in mortality rates throughout the span. The mean percent annual variation in diarrhoeal disease mortality, for most Latin American countries, indicates a marked decline in mortality (Fig. 1.2) (Mata 1983a). No definitive explanation is available for that behaviour, particularly because the trend was evident before the advent or oral rehydration. Greater information of the public about the nature and perils of diarrhoea, sustained improvements in income, education, nutrition, housing and hygiene, and gains in family planning and child spacing must have contributed to the declines in mortality in Cuba, Costa Rica, Jamica, Trinidad and Venezuela.

Diarrhoeal disease mortality is a main contributor to infant mortality, and both variables are highly correlated (Mata et al 1980). Therefore, if deaths due to diarrhoea decrease, so will infant deaths. This observation was clearly documented in Costa Rica (Mata 1983) permitting forecasts of fluctuations in infant mortality as a consequence of variations in diarrhoeal disease deaths. These observations provide further justification to emphasize control programes using the present knowledge on the epidemiology, aetiology and

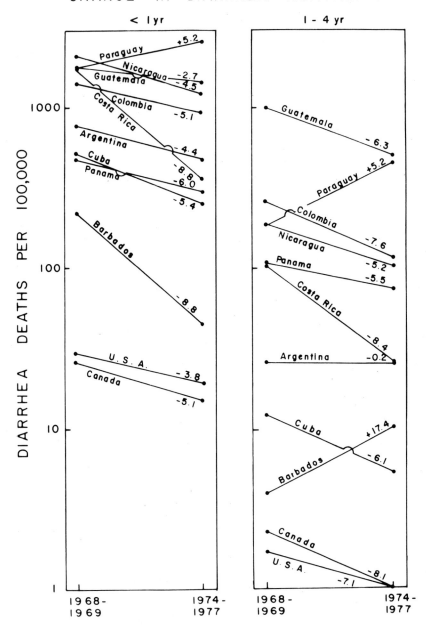

Fig. 1.2 Mortality due to diarrhoeal diseases, per 100 000 population, for infants and preschool children, selected countries of the Americas. The following should be noted: (a) marked differences in rates for the various countries; (b) consistent declines in mortality for most countries over the period 1968–69 to 1974–77. The mean per cent annual variation is shown next to the name of the country, and it generally negative, except for countries where a deterioration of diarrhoeal mortality appears to have occurred, for instance, in Paraguay and Barbados. The graph was prepared using official data published by the Pan American Health Organization (OPS 1980, WHO 1982).

treatment of the diarrhoeal diseases (Feachem & Koblinsky 1983, Feachem et al 1983, Mata 1983).

ACKNOWLEDGMENTS

Support was received from the University of Costa Rica, the World Health Organization and the National Council for Scientific Research and Technology.

REFERENCES

Barua D 1981 Diarrhea as a global problem and the WHO programme for its control. In: Holme T, Holmgren J, Merson M H, Mollby R (eds) Acute enteric infections in children. Elsevier/North Holland, Amsterdam, p 1–6

Béhar M, Ascoli W, Scrimshaw N S 1958 An investigation into the causes of death in children in four rural communities in Guatemala. Bulletin of the World Health Organization 19: 1093–1102

Black R E, Brown K H, Becker S, Yanus M 1982a Longitudinal studies of infectious diseases and physical growth of children in rural Bangladesh. I. Patterns of morbidity. American Journal of Epidemiology 115: 305–314

Black R E, Brown K H, Becker S, Alim A R M A, Huq I 1982b Longitudinal studies of infectious diseases and physical growth of children in rural Bangladesh. II. Incidence of diarrhoea and association with known pathogens. American Journal of Epidemiology 115: 315–324

Chen L C, Alauddin-Chowdhury A K M, Huffman S 1980 Anthropometric assessment of energy-protein malnutrition and subsequent risk of mortality among preschool aged children. American Journal of Clinical Nutrition 33: 1836–1845

Cole T J, Parkin J M 1977 Infection and its effects on the growth of young children: A comparison of The Gambia and Uganda. Transactions of the Royal Society of Tropical Medicine and Hygiene 71: 196–198

Feachem R G, Hogan R C, Merson M H 1983 Diarrhoeal disease control: reviews of potential interventions. Bulletin of the World Health Organization 61: 637–640

Feachem R G, Koblinsky M A 1983 Interventions for the control of diarrhoeal diseases among young children: measles immunization. Bulletin of the World Health Organization 61: 641–652

Field M 1976 Regulation of active ion transport in the small intestine. In: Elliott K, Knight J (eds) Acute diarrhoea in childhood. Ciba Foundation Symposium 42, Elsevier/Excerpta, Amsterdam, p 109–122

Gracey M, 1979 The contaminated small bowel syndrome. American Journal of Clinical Nutrition 32: 234–243

Lindebaum J, Gerson C D, Kent T H 1971 Recovery of small-intestinal structure and function after residence in the tropics. I. Studies in Peace Corp volunteers. Annals of Internal Medicine 74: 218–222

Martorell R, Yarbrough C, Yarbrough S, Klein R E 1980 The impact of ordinary illnesses on the dietary intakes of malnourished children. American Journal of Clinical Nutrition 33: 345–350

Mata L 1978 The Children of Santa Maria Cauqué. A prospective field study of health and growth. The MIT Press, Cambridge, Mass

Mata L 1979 The malnutrition-infection complex and its environment factors. Proceedings of the Nutrition Society 38: 29–40

Mata L 1982 Malnutrition and concurrent infections. Comparison of two populations with different infection rates. In: Mackenzie J S (ed) Viral diseases in South-East Asia and the Western Pacific. Academic Press, Australia, ch 7, p 56–76

Mata L 1983a Epidemiology of acute diarrhea in childhood. An overview. In: Bellanti J A (ed) Acute diarrhoea: its nutritional consequences in children. Nestlé, Vevey/Raven Press, New York, ch 1, p 3–22

Mata L 1983b Influence on the growth parameters of children. Comments. In: Bellanti J A (ed) Acute diarrhea: its nutritional consequences in children. Nestlé, Vevey/Raven Press, New York, p 85–94

Mata L 1983 The evolution of diarrhoeal diseases and malnutrition in Costa Rica. The role of interventions. Assignment Children 61/62: 195–224

Mata L, Kronmal R A, Villegas H 1980 Diarrhoeal diseases: a leading world health problem. In: Ouchterlony O, Holmgren J (eds) Cholera and related diarrhoeas. Molecular aspects of a global health problem, S Karger, Basel p 1–14

Mata L J, Urrutia J J, Gordon J E 1978 Diseases and disabilities. In: Mata L J (ed) The children of Santa Maria Cauqué. The MIT Press, Cambridge, ch 12, p 254–292

Mata L J, Urrutia J J, Lechtig A 1971 Infection and nutrition of children of a low socioeconomic rural community. American Journal of Clinical Nutrition 24: 249–259

Mata L, Urrutia J J, Simhon A 1984 Infectious agents in acute and chronic diarrhea of childhood. In: Lebenthal E (ed) Chronic diarrhea in children. Nesté, Vevey/Raven Press, New York, p 237–252

Mata L, Simhon A, Urrutia J J, Kronmal R A, Fernandez R, Garcia B 1983 Epidemiology of rotaviruses in a cohort of 45 Guatemalan Mayan Indian children observed from birth to the age of three years. Journal of Infectious Diseases 148: 452–461

Molla A M, Molla A, Sarker S A, Rahaman M M 1983a Food intake during and after recovery from diarrhea in children. In: Chen L C, Scrimshaw N S (eds) Diarrhea and malnutrition. Plenum Pub Co, New York, ch 7, p 113–123

Molla A, Molla A M, Sarker S A, Khatoon M, Rahaman M M 1983b Effects of acute diarrhea on absorption of macronutrients during disease and after recovery. In: Chen L C, Scrimshaw N S (eds) Diarrhea and malnutrition. Plenum Pub Co, New York, ch 9, p 143–154

Organización Panamericana de la Salud 1980 Enfermedades diarreicas en las Américas. Boletin Epidemiológico (PAHO), Washington DC, 1:1–4

Puffer R C, Serrano C V 1973 Patterns of mortality in childhood, PAHO Sci Pub No 262, PAHO, Washington DC

Rahaman M M, Wahed M A 1983 Direct nutrient loss and diarrhea. In: Chen L C, Scrimshaw N S (eds) Diarrhea and malnutrition. Plenum Pub Co, New York, ch 10, p 155–160

Rohde J E, Northrup R S 1976 Taking science where the diarrhoea is. In: Elliott K, Knight J (eds) Acute diarrhoea in childhood, Ciba Foundation Symposium 42, Elsevier/Excerpta, Amsterdam, p 339–358

Scrimshaw N S, Taylor C E, Gordon J E 1959 Interactions of nutrition and infection. American Journal of Medical Sciences 237: 367–403

Snyder J D, Merson M H 1982 The magnitude of the global problem of acute diarrhoeal disease: a review of active surveillance data. Bulletin of the World Health Organization 60: 605–613

Whitehead R G 1981 Malnutrition and infection. In: Isliker H, Scruch B (eds) The impact of malnutrition on immune defense in parasitic infestation. Hans Huber, Bern p 15–25

World Health Organization 1980 Scientific working group reports 1978–1980. Programme for Control of Diarrhoeal Diseases, CDD/80.1, WHO, Geneva

World Health Organization 1982 Diarrhoeal diseases control programme. An overview of the problem in America. Weekly Epidemiological Record 57: 353–360

World Health Organization 1983 Infant and young child nutrition. Report by the Director-General, Document A36/7, WHO, Geneva

Pathogenesis of diarrhoea

INTRODUCTION

Diarrhoea is a prominent clinical feature of childhood malnutrition and diarrhoeal illnesses are major causes of the high levels of childhood morbidity and mortality in malnourished populations. Diarrhoea can result from a vast array of underlying causes; these include inborn errors of metabolism, allergies, chemical irritation or osmotic overload in the intestine, systemic and idiopathic inflammatory diseases and hormone-secreting tumours. In children with malnutrition the overwhelming bulk of diarrhoeal episodes are due to gastrointestinal infections. The mechanisms involved in producing diarrhoea in such children form the subject matter for this chapter.

Over the past decade knowledge about the causes of infectious diarrhoeas has increased rapidly. This has resulted from technical developments in diagnostic microbiology which are being applied in epidemiological studies that are providing a clearer understanding of the causes of diarrhoeal diseases, particularly in developing countries where they are so prevalent. Examples of this new knowledge include the discovery that many diarrhoeal illnesses are due to viruses and enterotoxigenic bacteria which would not have been detected, or even sought, only 10 years ago.

The clinical setting for diarrhoeal diseases in malnourished children must be kept in mind. The usual background of poverty, ignorance, overcrowding and inadequate hygiene in tropical regions of the developing world or in disadvantaged minority groups in otherwise healthy societies tends to perpetuate the problem. In these circumstances multiple pathology, for example, involving the respiratory and gastrointestinal tracts, is the rule rather than the exception and coexisting diseases, like measles or malaria, are often associated with bouts of diarrhoea. Specific underlying gastrointestinal diseases, such as tuberculous enteritis, may also coexist and present only when complications, such as stricture or fistula formation, cause acute problems or when an acute intercurrent attack of gastroenteritis leads to diarrhoea and dehydration.

INTESTINAL FUNCTION AND MICROBIAL CONTROL MECHANISMS

Interactions among mirco-organisms and between them and the gastrointestinal mucosa are essential features of the intestinal 'microecology'. There are two main ways the ecological balance is disturbed in malnourished children with diarrhoeal disease:

1. Infections with pathogenic micro-organisms
2. Disturbances of the populations of indigenous micro-organisms.

The upper small intestine is involved with digestion and absorption of dietary nutrients which mix with secretions from salivary glands, stomach, biliary tree, pancreas and small amounts of intestinal secretions. In health, these contribute several litres daily which are conserved by being reabsorbed through the jejunum, ileum and colon with only small amounts being lost in faeces.

Apart from digestion and absorption of carbohydrates, fats and proteins, the small intestine is also involved in transfer of fluid and electrolyes (Dobbins & Binder 1981). Most intestinal transport, except passive non-ionic diffusion, is sodium linked. This is facilitated by the so-called sodium pump which is NA^+, K^+-ATPase dependent and which extrudes the ion at the basolateral membrane of the enterocyte; this helps maintain a low intracellular sodium (Na) concentration and a transcellular potential difference. Apical enterocytes have mechanisms for Na^+ coupled glucose and amino acid transport; there are also anion-cation exchange mechanisms. Crypt cells help achieve a secondary form of active luminal secretion of chloride ions and are considered not to be involved in Na^+coupled glucose and amino acid absorption.

Cyclic adenosine monophosphate (cAMP) normally helps regulate intestinal electrolyte transport by inhibiting Na^+: Cl^- influx, by stimulating active Cl^- secretion by increasing the permeability of the brush border membrane and by stimulating active HCO_3^- secretion. Cyclic guanidine mosophosphate (GMP) is also an intracellular mediator of electrolyte transport and is thought to induce active Cl^- secretion and probably inhibits Na^+: Cl^- influx. Calcium also has an important regulatory role and may be the mediator for cAMP-induced secretion. This involves the calcium-dependent regulatory protein, calmodulin, although the precise mechanisms are not known. These mechanisms are important because of their involvement in secretion induced by bacterial enterotoxins which are potent secretagogues.

Complex bacterial interactions help determine the composition of the 'relatively sterile' upper intestinal microflora and the normal bacterial and viral populations in the lumen deter the overgrowth of pathogens (Gracey 1982). Local secretory antibodies also help protect against adhesion of enteric pathogens to the intestinal mucosa, apparently by blocking specific binding sites on the bacterial cell wall and so inhibiting bacterial adherence to epithelial surfaces. The net effect of such protective measures is to deter colonisation and to increase the clearance of micro-organisms by the surface secretions. Intestinal antibodies also protect against toxic bacterial metabolites, such as enterotoxins. Secretory antitoxins are capable of complexing with exotoxins, such as cholera toxin, to prevent binding to mucosal receptors, thus interfering with activation of mucosal adenylate cyclase which mediates toxin induced net fluid and electrolyte secretion.

INFECTIONS WITH PATHOGENIC MICRO-ORGANISMS

Enterotoxigenic bacteria

Vibrio cholerae is the best known and most extensively studied enterotoxigenic micro-organism. The major steps by which it causes acute, watery diarrhoea are:

1. ingestion of a sufficiently large inoculum
2. passage and survival through the stomach (which is enhanced in subjects with hypochlorhydria)
3. multiplication in the alkaline environment of the upper intestinal lumen
4. elaboration of cholera toxin (CT)
5. binding of the exotoxin to the intestinal cell wall, which
6. stimulates intracellular adenylate cyclase activity, which
7. leads to increased intracellular concentrations of cyclic adenosine 3', 5' monophosphate (cAMP), which
8. are responsible for net transmucosal fluid and electrolyte secretion.

These actions are confined to the small intestine and occur despite the structural integrity of the intestinal mucosa being maintained. This helps explain why patients with cholera respond so completely to replacement of gastrointestinal fluid losses.

Enterotoxigenic *E. Coli* (ETEC)

Over the past few years enterotoxigenic bacteria have become recognized as important causes of infectious diarrhoeas. As Carpenter (1980) remarks: 'enterotoxigenic *E. coli* have proved to be a significant cause of acute diarrhoeal disease in almost every region where they have been seriously sought'. It is now becoming recognized that enterotoxigenicity is not confined to *Vibrio cholerae* and *E. coli*; this mechanism is common to several enteric pathogens and the list seems to be still expanding as appropriate epidemiological and laboratory investigations are undertaken (see Table 2.1).

The ability of enterotoxigenic bacteria to adhere to the gastrointestinal mucosa seems important in determining whether they are important enteric pathogens. With enterotoxigenic strains of *E. coli* (ETEC), for example, the presence of a colonization factor antigen (CFA) is needed to allow adhesion to occur (Evans & Evans 1978). Enterotoxigenic strains of *E. coli* produce

Table 2.1

Micro-organism	Initial events	Pathogenic mechanisms
V. cholerae	Adherence	Toxin stimulation of adenylate cyclase
Enterotoxigenic *E. coli*	Adherence	Toxin stimulation of adenylate cyclase (or guanylate cyclase by ST)
Enteropathogenic *E. coli*		Invasion, sometimes toxin production
Shigella	Invasion	Mucosal inflammation, destruction
Salmonella	Invasion	Inflammation, monocyte response
Campylobacter	Invasion	
Aeromonas	Adhesion or Invasion	Toxin production causing secretion (enterotoxin) and mucosal damage (cytotoxin)
Yersina	?	Toxin production, ? role
Clostridium difficile	?	Toxin production and local damage Ca^+-linked secretion
Giardia lamblia	Adhesion	Damage to enterocytes, malabsorption
Entamoeba hystolytica	Invasion	Invasion, inflammation, necrosis
Yeasts		Toxin production
Viruses	Invasion	Inflammation, mucosal damage and malabsorption

a heat-labile toxin (LT), a heat-stable toxin (ST) or both. LT is a large molecular weight toxin which is antigenically and physiologically related to cholera toxin (CT). It binds to GM1 ganglioside in the intestinal mucosal cell wall, although this binding is not so avid as with CT, it stimulates the secretion of isotonic fluid which persists after exposure to the mucosa. Like cholera toxin, LT is antigenic and there is some immunological cross-reactivity between the two toxins. The heat-stable toxin, ST, is a much smaller molecule, it does not bind gangliosides, is only weakly antigenic and appears to act by stimulating guanylate cyclase leading to increased intracellular levels of cyclic GMP in the intestinal mucosa. The effects of ST are gut-specific; they do not occur, for example, with liver, pancreas or stomach and the effects on the large intestine are much less than on the duodenum, jejunum or ileum.

LT blocks Na^+ and Cl^- absorption by villous epithelial cells and, simultaneously, induces Cl^- and HCO_3^- secretion by the crypt cells through the mediation of adenylate cyclase. ST acts through guanylate cyclase and has a similar action on villous cells but has much less influence on choride and bicarbonate secretion by the crypt cells which helps explain why ST-induced fluid losses are milder than with LT.

Some *E. coli* have entero-invasive properties like *Shigella* and cause a dysenteric type of diarrhoea. This may occur with other bacteria including *Campylobacter* and species of *Aeromonas*.

Enteropathogenic *E. coli* (EPEC)

There is some disagreement about the clinical importance of enteropathogenic *E. coli* (EPEC). There is good evidence that these are important in epidemics of diarrhoea in infants and young children (Rogers 1951), which was how they were initially recognized. However, most of these strains, which traditionally are identified by sero-typing, do not produce entero-toxins. The mechanisms by which they cause diarrhoea are uncertain although it is known that some strains produce a toxin similar to the toxin produced by *Shigella dysenteriae* type 1, the Shiga bacillus (O'Brien et al 1977). A strain of *E. coli*, O26: H11, has been shown to be adherent to an in vitro preparation of human fetal intestinal mucosa and this property is mannose resistant (McNeish et al 1975). EPEC strains from an outbreak of infantile diarrhoea have also been found to be adhesive in a HEp2 tissue culture system (Cravioto et al 1979). Patterns of haemagglutination (HA) typing of EPEC have also been linked to diarrhoea and HA typing, used in conjunction with sero-typing, has been proposed for their identification (Evans et al 1979). Some EPEC strains also possess a factor (VT) cytotoxic to Vero cells (Konowalchuk et al 1977) which is transferable to *E. coli* K12; the possible clinical significance of the VT factor is uncertain (Rowe 1981).

Enterotoxigenic strains of *E. coli* from different parts of the world are often of the same sero-type, including O6: H16, O8: H9, O15: H11, O25: H42, O78: H11 and O78: H12 (Orskov et al 1976). This has led to a renewed interest in identifying enterotoxigenic bacteria by sero-grouping. It has been proposed recently that most ETEC could be identified simply be sero-grouping, using polyvalent antisera selected from a range of sero-groups and sero-types corresponding to LT-producing and ST-producing strains of *E. coli* from several geographical regions (Merson et al 1980). Such a scheme has appeal as it would lessen the need for identification of toxigenic strains by more cumbersome means, such as the suckling mouse test for ST (Berry et al 1983b, Burke et al 1981) or the ELISA method for LT (Yolken et al 1977). The proposal by Merson and his colleagues was included in an epidemiological study of Aboriginal children in remote communities in the tropical North West of Australia (Berry et al 1983a). Toxin testing was done by the suckling mouse test and by ELISA and 58 ETEC strains were identified, 40 of them had either an H32 or an O126 antigen and only 3 out of the 58 stains would have been detected using the polyvalent sera proposed by Merson et al (1980). This may be because of geographical variations in distribution of toxigenic and pathogenic strains. Further studies need to be done in other geographical regions to test this system and regular checks need to be made to monitor shifts in distribution of *E. coli* strains.

Ulshen & Rollo (1980) recently studied, in some detail, an infant with diarrhoea associated with an EPEC (O125) which did not produce LT or ST and was not entero-invasive but penetrated the glycocalyx of the intestinal brush border membrane and caused extensive ultrastructural and histological damage to the mucosa; this suggests another mechanism for the production of diarrhoea by pathogenic strains of *E. coli*.

Other enterotoxigenic bacteria

In recent years other bacteria have been found to be enterotoxigenic, these including *Shigella dysenteriae* I, *Shigella flexneri*, *Staphylococcus aureus*, *Clostridium perfringens*, *Clostridium difficile*, *Pseudomonas aeruginosa*, *Yersinia enterolitica*, *Bacillus cereus*, *Klebsiella pneumoniae* and *Aeromonas* species (Thorne & Gorbach 1979). These and other bacteria, such as *Campylobacter*, are now recognized as important causes or diarrhoeal illnesses and they will not be detected in clinical and epidemiological studies unless special laboratory methods are used for their isolation and identification. A recently reported study from Perth has highlighted this.

A prospective 12-month long study of over 1000 children with acute diarrhoea was undertaken to determine the relative importance of *Aeromonas* species as a cause of childhood gastroenteritis (Gracey et al 1982). This was combined with methods to detect ETEC, *Salmonella*, *Shigella*, *Campylobacter* and rotavirus (Burke et al 1983). Enterotoxigenic *Aeromonas* species were the most frequently recognized bacterial cause of diarrhoea being isolated in over 10 per cent of patients, in comparison, for example, with ETEC in 2 per cent campylobacter in 7.4 per cent and salmonella in 5.7 per cent. *Aeromonas* spp. are easily confused with enterobacteria unless oxidase testing is done routinely. Our hospital's diagnostic mocrobiology laboratory now routinely look for aeromonas in faecal specimens by growing them on an ampicillin-enriched blood agar medium on which they appear as flat greyish colonies often surrounded by a zone of β-haemolysis. Enterotoxigenic strains can easily be detected, with 97 per cent accuracy, by a simple, in vitro haemolysin assay (Burke et al 1981). A recent editorial comment suggests that *Aeromonas* gastroenteritis may be an important cause of diarrhoea throughout the world and emphasizes the importance of awareness of this organism and the use of appropriate laboratory methods for its identification (Editorial, 1983).

Shigella

Strains of *Shigella* cause clinical disease after invading the intestinal wall, causing inflammation and tissue destruction. Characteristically, patients with shigellosis are systemically ill with high fever, watery, blood-stained diarrhoea with mucus, and often have abdominal pain and vomiting. The infection becomes established first in the small intestine and later extends to the colon where mucosal invasion causes urgency, tenesmus, and bloody, mucous diarrhoeal stools which are frequent but smaller than in the earlier phase of the disease.

Salmonella

Salmonella strains are also invasive and penetrate into the lamina propria and can become blood-borne and travel to other tissues, such as joints or the central nervous system. In most cases the infection and inflammation are confined to the gut and are associated with diarrhoea and vomiting.

Viruses

A detailed discussion about the viral diarrhoeas is given by Lam and Madeley elsewhere in this book (see Ch. 5). The Norwalk and Hawaii viruses which have been associated with epidemics of gastroenteritis of small to very large scale (Blacklow & Cukor, 1981) produce patchy, histological damage in the proximal small intestine in humans which clears within two weeks. The gastric and large intestinal mucosa is unaffected. The small intestinal lesion is associated with impaired xylose and fat absorption and lowered disaccharidase activity although adenylate cyclase activity is normal (Levy et al 1976).

Human rotavirus particles were first detected in duodenal biopsy specimens which showed patchy irregularities of the mucosal surface with shortening and blunting of the villi and extensive damage to the microvilli which was associated with depressed disaccharidase activity (Bishop et al 1973). Similar findings have been made since by many other groups of workers. The human rotavirus selectively damages the apical parts of duodenal and upper jejunal mucosa but not the other parts of the gastrointestinal tract. The pathophysiology of transmissable gastroenteritis (TGE) of piglets, which closely resembles human rotavirus enteritis, shows the virus rapidly invades the villous enterocytes, but not the crypt enterocytes, before diarrhoea occurs (Shepherd et al 1979). Later, histological damage causes impaired brush border enzyme activities (disaccharidases and Na^+, and K^+ ATPase) and at the height of the diarrhoea, rapid enterocyte turnover leads the small intestinal mucosa to consist mostly of immature, undifferentiated cells with short, blunt villi and relatively deep crypts.

Characteristically, rotavirus infections are accompanied by severe watery diarrhoea with fever, vomiting, dehydration and metabolic acidosis. The stools usually contain higher than normal concentrations of sodium and chloride and variable amounts of sugar (Tallett et al 1977, Nalin et al 1978). Molla et al (1981) have shown that faecal losses of sodium and bicarbonate are much less than in ETEC diarrhoea or cholera and the chloride concentration in stools slighly less than with ETEC and less than one-third that in cholera stools (see Table 2.2).

Table 2.2   Stool electrolytes in acute childhood diarrhoea (from Molla et al 1981)

Cause of diarrhoea	Stool electrolytes (mmol/l)				mmols
	Na^+	K^+	Cl^-	HCO_3^-	
Rotavirus	37	38	22	6	300
Cholera	88	30	86	32	300
ETEC	53	37	24	18	300
WHO rehydration solution	90	20	80	30	330

This suggests that the widely recommended World Health Organization (WHO) oral rehydration formula may not be appropriate for treatment of rotavirus diarrhoea. This is mostly a disease of infants and children below 24 months and diarrhoea tends to start later and last longer than the vomiting; episodes may be accompanied or preceded by a respiratory illness.

Yeasts

Little is known of the possible role of yeasts in childhood gastroenteritis. Malnourished children have an impaired ability to kill yeasts (Tuck et al 1979) and this may help explain why species of *Candida*, particularly the pathogens *C. albicans*, *C.parpasilosis* and *C. tropicalis* are increased significantly in their upper gastrointestinal secretions (Gracey et al 1974). Children with chronic diarrhoea have defective yeast opsonization (Candy et al 1980) and overgrowth of *C. albicans* in the upper gut of infants with gastroenteritis has been associated with depression of duodenal lactase activity (Barnes et al 1974) suggesting it may play a part in mucosal damage and disaccharidase deficiency, perhaps on top of mucosal injury initiated by viruses or other infections agents. It has also been shown that some *Candida* species, including *C. albicans* and *C. tropicalis*, have toxin-like effects in experimental animals (Thelen et al 1978) and may contribute to net intestinal fluid loss and carbohydrate malabsorption in acute gastroenteritis.

Parasites

Malnourished children with diarrhoeal diseases commonly have parasitic gut infections but is is often difficult to ascribe a causal pathogenic role for the parasites in the clinical picture of the diarrhoeal illness. The patterns of parasitic infections have great geographical diversity (see Ch. 6) and in many regions *Giardia lamblia* and *Entamoeba histolytica* are associated with acute or chronic diarrhoeal illnesses caused by heavy intestinal parasitosis and mucosal tissue damage and destruction; these may be so extensive as to cause intestinal malabsorption. In some regions, especially in the tropics, intestinal invasion and blood loss caused by parasites such as *Ancylostoma duodenale* (hookworm) are causes of chronic and sometimes profound anaemia which is an important part of the clinical syndrome of the diarrhoea-malnutrition cycle. Parasitic gut infections are sometimes so heavy as to present with acute, watery diarrhoea or they may be so chronic and/or intermittent as to cause a chronic malabsorption syndrome which may only become inportant when an intercurrent, acute gastrointestinal infection leads to an episode of diarrhoea and dehydration.

Mucosal pathology

The high frequency of bacterial, viral and parasitic gut infections in malnourished children is associated with repeated or chronic episodes of damage to the upper small intestinal mucosa. Malnutrition, itself, is associated with subclinical small intestinal disease and impaired epithelial cell renewal causes widespread structural abnormalities in the gut mucosa. Even apparently healthy adults living in the tropics have altered gastrointestinal morphology with shorter, wider villi and with irregular enterocytes and inflammatory cell infiltration in the lamina propria in comparison with Western control subjects (Sprinz et al 1962). In malnourished children the histological abnormalities in the proximal small intestinal mucosa are quite severe; they include thinning of the gut wall, marked flattening and broadening of the villi, extensive inflammation in the lamina propria and transformation of the epithelial cells from columnar to squamous. The severity and type of malnutrition (e.g. kwashiorkor or marasmus) has some influence on these changes with the changes in kwashiorkor being much worse because of protein deprivation damaging cellular replication and renewal in the crypts of Lieberkühn (Brunser 1977). The gastric mucosa is also damaged and gastric acid secretion impaired, predisposing the gut to overgrowth by micro-organisms.

The severe and extensive histological damage in the upper intestinal mucosa which occurs in malnourished children is associated with impaired brush border enzyme activities, e.g. disaccharidases and peptidases, which contribute to impaired digestion and absorption of nutrients. Mucosal changes can be so serious as to lead to protein-losing enteropathy. Steatorrhoea also occurs and has been related to impaired micelle formation due to depletion of the bile salt pool (Schneider & Viteri 1974) although depressed exocrine pancreatic secretions causing decreased intraluminal lipolysis (Blackburn & Vinijchaikul 1969) or defective β-lipoprotein production for transport of fat into lymph could also be involved.

MICROBIAL CONTAMINATION OF THE UPPER GUT

Bacterial contamination of upper intestinal secretions has been found in malnourished children in Central America, Africa, Asia and in Australian Aborigines (Gracey 1981). Normally, the upper intestinal contents are kept 'relatively sterile' (i.e. $<10^3$ to 10^4 micro-organisms per ml) by a combination of controlling influences which include secretion of hydrochloric acid by the gastric mucosa, the cleansing effect of gut peristalsis (the 'intestinal housekeeper'), the 'trap-door' action of the ileocaecal valve which limits proximal contamination by the normally profuse colonic microflora, immunological factors and the presence of bile salts in the intestinal juice (Gracey 1979). In malnutrition several of these mechanisms may be impaired, e.g. gastric secretion, immunological responses and gut motility, predisposing to uncontrolled bacterial contamination in the upper gut which is made much more likely by living in grossly contaminated environments and by being exposed to faecally contaminated food, water and eating and drinking utensils (Rowland & McCollum 1977).

Clinical effects

Upper intestinal bacterial contamination can cause a range of clinical effects including diarrhoea and malabsorption and this is likely to be important in children with malnutrition and diarrhoeal diseases. Steatorrhoea is related to degradation of bile salts which reduces their intraluminal concentration to below the critical micellar concentration which thus prevents efficient micellar solubilization of lipid and causes malabsorption of fat (Tabaqchali et al 1968). Upper intestinal bacterial overgrowth can cause carbohydrate malabsorption by the damaging effects of bacterially deconjugated bile salts on metabolically dependent active transport mechanisms in the enterocytes which line the intestinal epithelium. Carbohydrate malabsorption can be a serious clinical problem in malnutrition, particularly in severely malnourished infants and young children in whom it can cause severe, life-threatening diarrhoea, hypoglycaemia and metabolic acidosis and a temporary inability to absorb all carbohydrates including glucose, galactose and fructose (Lifshitz et al 1970). Carbohydrate malabsorption in this situation may also be contributed to by the effects of enterotoxins on transmucosal transport (Thelen et al 1978) as well as the bile salt-mediated mechanisms. Upper intestinal overgrowth by toxigenic micro-organisms, such as *Klebsiella*, *Proteus*, *Shigella* and staphylococci, may also contribute to toxin-induced net fluid and electrolyte secretion although those bacteria are not generally regarded as 'enteropathogenic' (Thelen et al 1978). Bacterial overgrowth causes other absorptive defects including impaired amino acid absorption and malabsorption of vitamin B_{12}.

The mucosal lesion

Upper intestinal bacterial contamination also has significant effects on the ultrastructural integrity of the small intestinal mucosa. This extensive, patchy damage to the mucosa is not caused by bacterial invasion and has been considered due to the toxic effects of unconjugated bile salts. However, other causative factors related to byproducts of bacterial metabolism have been invoked; these include bacterial exotoxins, alcohol and short-chain fatty acids injurious to the intestinal mucosa (Giannella et al 1974). Fatty acids produced by bacterial hydroxylation (e.g. ricinoleic acid, the active principle of castor oil) appear to be able to impair sodium and water absorption and to impair intestinal motility and increase mucus secretion (Phillips 1972). Bile acid malabsorption can also contribute to steatorrhoea and diarrhoea by impairing colonic water reabsorption

It has been suggested that bacterial proteases may be responsible for damage to the brush border in conditions of bacterial overgrowth. Jonas et al (1978) showed a bacterial protease in experimentally induced overgrowth, perhaps a bacterial elastase, which releases disaccharidases from the brush border. *Bacteroides* is able to produce proteases which depress human brush border sucrase and maltase activities, although many other bacterial species, including *Clostridium* spp., anaerobic lactobacilli, *E. coli*, *Klebsiella* spp. and *Proteus* spp. seems to lack this capability (Riepe et al, 1980). It is possible that several of these mechanisms act simultaneously to produce mucosal damage and impaired mucosal digestion and intestinal transport of important nutrients including sugars and amino acids and, perhaps, secretion of fluid and electrolytes in the presence of upper gut contamination.

POST-ENTERITIS DIARRHOEA

Mucosal damage associated with acute and recurrent gastrointestinal infections sometimes causes a 'post-gastroenteritis' syndrome characterized by diarrhoea, malabsortpion and failure to thrive without any obvious infectious cause. Secondary sugar intolerance is an important cause of relapse after episodes of gastroenteritis, particularly in poorly nourished infants and young children. Lactose intolerance is the commonest form of secondary sugar intolerance and is caused by depression of lactase activity consequent on damage to the intestinal mucosa; other disaccharidases, such as sucrase, may also be depressed although this is rarely of clinical importance. In severely malnourished individuals temporary monosaccharide malabsorption may cause an intolerance to all carbohydrates including the monosaccharides glucose, galactose and fructose. These secondary forms of sugar intolerance are common and cause an osmotic type of diarrhoea and dehydration with fluid, acidic stools containing excessive amounts of sugars which can be detected in fresh faecal specimens as reducing substances. Appropriate dietary manipulations and supportive therapy should effectively manage secondary sugar intolerance (Anderson & Burke 1975).

Other patients appear to be intolerant of milk proteins after gastrointestinal infections, perhaps because of intestinal damage and permeability sensitizing them to foreign proteins. These patients usually have diarrhoea, sometimes with blood and mucus, vomiting and may have wheezing and recurrent respiratory infections. Attempts have been made lately to detect this disorder by immunological criteria such as raised serum IgA, serum precipitins to cow's milk, increased serum complement C3 and C4, raised serum IgE and skin testing, but none of these can replace adequately conducted challenge tests (Yadav & Iyngkaran 1981) as adequate diagnostic tests. Peroral biopsy has been used to document this condition but this procedure should not be undertaken lightly as a routine diagnostic test, particulary as many of the histological features are non-specific. Secondary intolerance to other foreign proteins (e.g. in soy, egg, chicken or goat's milk) has also been reported (Vitoria et al 1982) so dietary exclusion therapy can be very complicated and should not be undertaken without strong clinical indications.

NON-SPECIFIC, PRESUMED INFECTIOUS DIARRHOEAS

Despite extensive investigations, a significant proportion of infants and young children with presumed infectious diarrhoea have no identifiable cause for their illness. Some of these may be caused by 'newer' bacterial or viral agents which will not be detected unless special methods are used; some may be caused by agents which are not yet discovered or recognizable with currently available techniques and cause diarrhoea through pathogenic mechanisms as yet unknown.

Burke et al (1965) studied 12 babies with 'refractory diarrhoea' after an illness typical of acute gastroenteritis; 9 patients had multiple intestinal biopsies performed. All patients had sugar intolerance when they had diarrhoea and their initial biopsies showed various degrees of histological damage with shortened, blunted villi and inflammatory cell infiltration in the underlying lamina propria. Activities of mucosal enzymes, particularly lactase, were depressed and diarrhoea improved after lactose was removed from the diet; the mucosal abnormalities and enzyme activities returned to normal after 1 to 18 months. Many subsequent reports have confirmed temporary mucosal damage and depression of mucosal disaccharidases in similar patients which helps explain how secondary sugar intolerance caused 'refractory' diarrhoea in children following episodes of acute gastroenteritis.

Barnes & Townely (1973) made similar observations in 31 children with gastroenteritis and, in a later study, found overgrowth of upper intestinal secretions by *Candida albicans* in patients with lowered lactase activity (Barnes et al 1974). Zoppi et al (1977) found mucosal damage with clubbing and shortening of villi with mild to severe infiltration of the lamina propria by lymphocytes and plasma cells in a group of infants with 'persistent post-enteritis diarrhoea'. Our understanding of the pathogenesis of infections diarrhoeas is improving with the discoverey of previously unrecognized mechanisms, such as the actions of bacterial enterotoxins on the intestinal mucosa.

One of the virulence mechanisms of enterotoxigenic bacteria is the production of a colonization factor antigen (CFA) which facilitates adherence of bacteria to the intestinal mucosa. Candy et al (1981) used a buccal epithelial cell (BEC) assay to study an outbreak of acute diarrhoea in children. An adhesive strain of *E. coli* (O1: K1: H7) adhered significantly more frequently to BEC from infants with protracted diarrhoea than from children with acute diarrhoea, healthy infants and healthy adults. Enterobacteria from patients with protracted diarrhoea were also found to be more likely to adhere to their own BEC than to BEC from healthy adults. Enterocytes from patients with protracted diarrhoea were also more adhesive and this may help explain why bacterial overgrowth of the upper intestinal secretions is common in infants with protracted diarrhoea.

The recent case report by Ulshen & Rollo (1980), already discussed in relation to EPEC, has shows how some *E. coli* which are not invasive or enterotoxigenic may damage the gastrointestinal mucosa by adhering to it and thus causing villous blunting and inflammatory infiltration in the lamina propria. This mechanism may have been operating in patients with protracted diarrhoea mentioned above and this and other undefined mechanisms might help explain otherwise unexplained episodes of childhood diarrhoeal illnesses.

SUMMARY

Diarrhoea is a prominent clinical feature of childhood malnutrition and is mostly due to gastrointestinal infections and infestations. These are often caused by multiple pathogens and are commonly associated with infections in other organ systems, notably the respiratory tract.

Mechanisms causing diarrhoea in malnourished children can be grouped into those associated with structural damage to the intestinal mucosa and those due to changes in the intraluminal environment. Structural damage occurs, characteristically, with entro-invasive bacteria and with enteric viruses. Bacteria which produce enterotoxins, such as *Vibrio cholerae* and enterotoxigenic *E. coli* (ETEC), cause intestinal fluid secretion which is stimulated by the enterotoxins and mediated by enzymatic processes within the enterocytes. Microbial contamination of the upper intestinal secretions is a feature of childhood malnutrition and has damaging effects on intestinal digestion and absorption. The intestinal mucosa, itself, is extensively damaged in children with malnutrition and this contributes to the diarrhoea — malnutrition cycle.

ACKNOWLEDGEMENTS
Work in the author's department is supported by the TVW Telethon Foundation, the National Health and Medical Research Council (of Australia), the Wellcome Trust and Nestlé Nutrition, S.A.

REFERENCES

Anderson C M, Burke V 1975 Disorders of Carbohydrate digestion digestion and absorption. In: Anderson C M Burke V (eds) Paediatric gastrogenterology. Blackwell Scientific Publications, Oxford, P 199–218
Barnes G L, Bishop R F, Townley R R W 1974 Microbial flora and disaccharidase depression in infantile gastroenteritis. Acta paediatrica Scandinavica 63: 423–426
Barnes G L, Townley R R W 1973 Duodenal mucosal damage in 31 infants with gastroenteritis. Archives of Disease in Childhood 48: 343–349
Berry R J, Bettelheim K A, Gracey M 1983a Studies on entero toxigenic *Escherichia coli* isolated from persons without diarrhoea in Western Australia. Journal of Hygiene (Camb) 88: 99–106
Berry R J, Burke V, Gracey M 1983b A modified infant mouse assay for bacterial enterotoxins. Transactions of the Royal Society of Tropical Medicine and Hygiene 77: 699–701
Bishop R F, Davidson G P, Homes I H, Ruck B J 1973 Virus particles in epithelial cells of duodenal mucosa from children with acute non-bacterial gastroenteritis. Lancet ii: 1281–1283

Blackburn W R, Vinijchaikul K 1969 The pancreas in kwashiorkor. An electron microscopic study. Laboratory Investigation 20: 305–318

Blacklow N R, Cukor G 1981 Viral gastroenteritis. New England Journal of Medicine 304: 397–406

Brunser O 1977 Effects of malnutrition on intestinal structure and function in children. Clinical Gastroenterology 6: 341–353

Burke V, Gracey M, Robinson J, Peck D, Beaman J, Bundell C 1983 The microbiology of childhood gastroenteritis: Aeromonas species and other infective agents. Journal of Infections Diseases 148: 68–74

Burke V, Kerry K R, Anderson C M 1965 The relationship of dietary lactose to refractory diarrhoea in infancy. Australian Paediatric Journal 1: 147–160

Burke V, Robinson J, Berry R J, Gracey M 1981 Detection of enterotoxins of Aeromonas hydrophila by a suckling mouse test. Journal of Medical Microbiology 14: 401–408

Candy D C A, Leung T S M, Phillips A D, Harries J T, Marshall W C 1981 Models for studying the adhesion of enterobacteria to the mucosa of the human intestinal tract. In: Adhesion and micro-organism pathogenicity. Ciba Foundation Symposium 80, Pitman Medical, Tunbridge Wells, p 79–83

Candy D C A, Larcher V F, Tripp J H, Harries J T, Harvey B A M, Soothill J F 1980 Yeast opsonisation in children with chronic diarrhoeal states. Archives of Disease in Childhood 55: 189–193

Carpenter C C J 1980 Clinical and pathophysiological features of diarrhea caused by Vibrio cholerae and Escherichia coli. In: Field M, Fordtran J S, Schultz S G (eds) Secretory diarrhea. American Physiological Society, Bethesda, Md. USA

Cravioto A, Gross R J, Scotland S M et al 1979 An adhesive factor found in strains of Escherichia coli belonging to the traditional infantile enteropathogenic serotypes Current Microbiology 3:95–99

Dobbins J W, Binder H J 1981 Pathophysiology of diarrhea: alterations in fluid and electrolyte transport. Clinical Gastroenterology 10: 605–625

Editorial 1983 Aeromonas hydrophila: An important cause of diarrhea? Gastroenterology 85: 1444–1445

Evans D G, Evans D J 1978 New surface-associated heat-labile colonisation factor antigen (CFA/II) produced by enterotoxigenic Escherichia coli of serogroups O6 and O8. Infection and Immunity 21: 638–647

Evans D J, Evans D G, Dupont H L 1979 Hemagglutination patterns of enterotoxigenic and enteropathogenic Escherichia coli determined with human, bovine, chicken, guinea pig erythrocytes in the presence and absence of mannose. Infection and Immunity 23: 336–346

Giannella R A, Rout W R, Toskes P P 1974 Jejunal brush border injury and impaired sugar and amino acid uptake in the blind loop syndrome. Gastroenterology 67: 965–974

Gracey M 1979 The contaminated small bowel syndrome: pathogenesis diagnosis and treatment. American Journal of Clinical Nutrition 32: 234–243

Gracey M S 1981 Nutrition, bacteria and the gut. British Medical Bulletin 37: 71–75

Gracey M 1982 Intestinal microflora and bacterial overgrowth in early life. Journal of Pediatric Gastroenterology and Nutrition 1: 13–22

Gracey M, Burke V, Robinson J, 1982 Aeromonas-associated gastroenteritis. Lancet ii: 1304–1306

Gracey M, Stone D E, Suharjono, Sunoto 1974 Isolation of Candida species from the gastrointestinal tract in malnourished children. American Journal of clinical Nutrition 27: 345–349

Jonas A, Krishnan C, Forstner G 1978 Pathogenesis of mucosal injury in the blind loop syndrome. Gastroenterology 75: 791–795

Konowalchuk J, Speir J I, Stavric S 1977 Vero response to a cytoxin of Escherichia coli. Infection and Immunity 18: 775–779

Levy A G, Widerlite L, Schwartz C J, Dolin R, Blacklow N R, Gardney J D, et al 1976 Jejunal adenylate cyclase activity in human subjects during viral gastroenteritis. Gastroenterology 70: 321–325

Lifshitz F, Coello-Ramirez P, Gutierres-Topete G 1970 Monosaccharide intolerance and hypoglycemia in infants with diarrhoea. I. Clinical course of 23 infants. Journal of Pediatrics 77: 595–603

McNeish A S, Turner P, Fleming J, Evans N 1975 Mucosal adherence of human enteropathogenic *Escherichia coli*. Lancet ii: 946–948

Merson M H, Rowe B, Black R E, Huq I, Glass R I, Eusof A 1980 Use of antisera for identification of enterotoxigenic *Escherichia coli*. Lancet ii: 222–224

Molla A M, Rahman M, Sarker S A, Sack D A, Molla A 1981 Stool electrolyte content and purging rates in diarrhoea caused by rotavirus, enterotoxigenic *E. coli*, and *V. cholerae* in children. Journal of Pediatrics 98: 835–838

Nalin D R, Levine M M, mata L, Cespedes C, Vargas W, Lizano C, et al 1978 Comparison of sucrose with glucose in oral therapy of infant diarrhoea. Lancet ii: 276–283

O'Brien A D, Thompson M R, Cantey J R, Formal S B 1977 Production of a *Shigella dysenteriae*-like toxin by pathogenic *Escherichia coli*. Federation Proceedings, Abstracts of Annual Meeting, p 32

Orskov F, Orskov I, Evans D R Jr, Sack R B, Sack D A, Wadstrom T 1976 Special *Escherichia coli* serotypes among enterotoxigenic strains from diarrhoea in adults and children. Medical Microbiology and Immunology 162: 73–80

Phillips S F 1972 Diarrhea: a current view of the pathophysiology. Gastroenterology 63: 495–518

Riepe S P, Goldstein J, Alpers D H 1980 Effect of secreted bacteroides proteases on human intestinal brush border hydrolases. Journal of Clinical Investigation 66: 314–322

Rogers K B 1951 The spread of infantile enteritis in a cubicle ward. Journal of Hygiene (Camb) 49: 140

Rowe B 1981 Enteropathogenic *Eschericia coli* (EPEC) — importance and pathophysiology. In: Holme T, Holmgren J, Merson M H, Möllby R (eds) Acute enteric infections in children. New prospects for treatment and prevention. Elsevier/North-Holland Biomedical Press, Amsterdam, p 101–106

Rowland M G M, McCollum J P K 1977 Malnutrition and gastroenteritis in the Gambia. Transactions of the Royal Society of Tropical Medicine and Hygiene 71: 199–203

Schneider R E, Viteri F E 1974 Luminal events of lipid absorption in protein-calorie malnourished children; relationship with nutritional recovery and diarrhea. I. Capacity of the duodenal content to achieve micellar solubilization of lipids. American Journal of Clinical Nutrition 27: 777–787

Shepherd R W, Butler D G, Cutz E, Gall D G, Hamilton J R 1979 The mucosal lesion in viral enteritis. Extent and dynamics of the epithelial response to virus invasion in transmissable gastroenteritis of piglets. Gastroenterology 76: 770–777

Sprinz H, Sribhibhadh R, Gangarosa E J, Benyajati C, Kundee D, Halstead S 1962 Biopsy of small bowel of Thai people. American Journal of Clinical Pathology 38: 43–51

Tabqchali S, Hatzioannou J, Booth C C 1968 Bile salt deconjugation and steatorrhoea in patients with the stagnant loop syndrome. Lancet ii: 12–16

Tallett S, MacKenzie C, Middleton P, Kerzner B, Hamilton R 1977 Clinical, laboratory, and epidemiological features of a viral gastroenteritis in infants and children. Pediatrics 60: 217–222

Thelen P, Burke V, Gracey M 1978 Effects of intestinal micro-organisms on fluid and electrolyte transport in the jejunum of the rat. Journal of Medical Microbiology 11: 463–470

Thorne G M, Gorbach S L 1979 New bacterial enterotoxins and human diarrheal diseases. In: Janowitz H D, Sachar D B (eds) Frontiers of knowledge in the diarrheal diseases. Projects in Health Inc, Upper Montclair, N J, USA, p 165–176

Tuck R, Burke V, Gracey M, Malajczuk A, Sunoto 1979 Defective Candida killing in childhood malnutrition. Archives of Disease in Childhood 54: 445–447

Ulshen M H, Rollo J L 1980 Pathogenesis of *Escherichia coli* gastroenteritis in man — another mechanism. New England Journal of Medicine 302: 99–101

Vitoria J C, Camanero C, Sojo A, Ruiz A, Rodriguez-Soriano J 1982 Enteropathy related to fish, rice and chicken. Archives of Disease in Childhood 57: 44–48

Yadav M, Iyngkaran N 1981 Immunological studies in cows' milk protein-sensitive enteropathy. Archives of Disease in Childhood 56: 24–30

Yolken R H, Greenberg H B, Merson M H, Sack R B, Kapikian A Z *Escherichia coli* heat-labile enterotoxin. Journal of Clinical Microbiology 6: 439–444

Zoppi G, Deganello A, Gaburro D 1977 Persistent post-enteritis diarrhea. European Journal of Pediatrics 126: 225–236

Altered gastrointestinal immunity in malnourished children

A definition and explanation of malnutrition is essential before the subject of altered gastrointestinal immunity in malnourished children is considered. In addition, normal gastrointestinal immune function during infancy and childhood must be described, emphasizing changes which occur with age. Only then is it possible to begin to establish a clear understanding of how malnutrition during childhood affects immune function of the gastrointestinal tract.

MALNUTRITION

Prevalence

Recent evidence suggests that factors operating before birth may lead to prematurity and/or a decreased birth weight (Viteri 1981). Premature and low birth weight infants have a greater risk of malnutrition and early death than full-term, well-nourished newborns (Viteri 1981). The frequency with which a child develops infectious diseases is determined in many instances by the presence of undernutrition (Scrimshaw 1975). But the prevalence of undernutrition in a population is influenced not only by the frequency of prematurity and infectious diseases, but also by the availability of food, poor environmental conditions, ignorance of optimal childhood nutrition, and unstable socioeconomic and political circumstances.

Protein-energy malnutrition (PEM) is a condition that is not confined to underdeveloped countries. An examination of 300 randomly picked pre-school children of poor black families in Memphis, Tennessee (United States), showed that about 18 per cent were below the third percentile of standards for weight and height, 25 per cent were anaemic, 27 per cent had retarded skeletal development, and 44 per cent had low levels of vitamin A (Zee et al 1970). In another study, Merritt & Suskind (1979) reported evidence of acute malnutrition in 30 per cent of an inpatient population of a large children's hospital in Boston.

Types

Protein-energy malnutrition is not a discrete, all-or-none phenomenon but rather an entity that spans an entire spectrum, ranging from subclinical malnutrition to lethal nutritional deficiency states (Suskind 1975). It is now recognized that a pure deficiency of a single nutrient rarely occurs. Vitamin and mineral deficiencies accompany those of protein and calories and, more importantly, there are interactions among these deficiencies.

Malnutrition may be classified as primary or secondary. Classically, children with primary malnutrition have an inadequate nutrient intake. Secondary malnutrition is present when nutrient intake appears adequate but nutrient needs and/or losses are excessive as a result of the primary disease state.

Malnourished children may also be classified as having marasmus (non-oedematous PEM), kwashiorkor (oedematous PEM), or marasmus-kwashiorkor. Children who have been completely starved develop marasmus. They lack dietary protein, calories, vitamins and minerals and ultimately develop the clinical picture of starvation. Marasmus generally develops over several weeks or months, whereas kwashiorkor often develops very acutely. The child at risk for developing kwashiorkor, prior to an acute infectious illness, in many instances may not be nutritionally differentiated from his/her siblings. With the onset of an infectious disease, the infant goes into negative nitrogen balance and kwashiorkor rapidly becomes apparent (Suskind 1975).

Malnutrition varies in severity. Gomez and coworkers (1955) developed criteria for defining first, second, and third degree malnutrition by comparing children against locally derived growth standards. First degree malnutrition was defined as a body weight between 75 to 90 per cent of the mean weight for age, second degree malnutrition as 60 to 75 per cent of the mean weight of age, and third degree malnutrition or marasmus, was defined as anything less than 60 per cent of the mean weight for age. Children with kwashiorkor (oedema and hypoalbuminaemia) were considered to have third degree malnutrition.

More recently, Waterlow (1972, 1973) stressed the importance of determining a child's deficit in weight for height, and height for age using the 50th percentile of the Harvard Standard. Children with deficits in weight for height are considered to have evidence of acute malnutrition. Those with height for age deficits suffer from chronic malnutrition and are considered to be growth retarded. Children may be both acutely and chronically malnourished. It is important to underscore that the severity (1st, 2nd, or 3rd degree) and chronicity of the undernourished state as well as the presence of infection interact to affect gastrointestinal immunity. It is difficult, if not impossible, to control for these variables in studies of human malnutrition and gastrointestinal immunity. Therefore, data often appear to be contradictory.

IMMUNE FUNCTION OF THE GASTROINTESTINAL TRACT

Immune protection in vertebrates is provided by a dual system that maintains two basic defences against foreign substances (toxins, antigens) and invaders (viruses, bacteria, parasites) (Udall & Walker 1983). Although both systems can potentially respond specifically to foreign substances, one response seems to predominate in any given situation. One system, the humoral immune system, is mediated through antibodies synthesized by B lymphocytes. Individual B cells, when activated by recognition of a foreign invader, differentiate into plasma cells, which secrete antibodies that bind specifically to foreign substances and bacteria, and initiate a variety of elimination responses. The second system, the cellular immune system, is primarily mediated by T lymphocytes. It is particularly effective against fungi, parasites, intracellular viral infections, cancer cells, and foreign tissue. The two systems, which provide overlapping protection, interact and are to some extent interdependent. However, they require additional cells and substances to function normally. In addition to B lymphocytes and T lymphocytes, the macrophage, a non-lymphoid accessory cell, is important to immune function, as are components of complement and lymphokines. These immune components are present in the intestinal tract and at other locations in the body and operate to protect the developing infant. Their presence throughout the entire gastrointestinal tract is necessary because the gut is the first site in the infant and child to come in contact with a variety of infectious, antigenic and toxic substances.

Gastrointestinal associated lymphoid tissues

Organized aggregates of lymphocytes, collectively termed the gastrointestinal associated lymphoid tissues (GALT), are present in the gastrointestinal tract. The most frequently cited examples of GALT are the tonsils, Peyer's patches, and the appendix. The aggregated lymphoid structures are generally considered the principal sites in the mucosa for interaction between antigen from the gut lumen and circulating lymphocytes, whereas the cells in the lamina propria and epithelium are the effector cells that mediate immune responses (Ottaway et al 1979).

Gastrointestinal associated lymphoid tissues have many features in common with either secondary or peripheral lymphoid tissues such as the spleen and lymph nodes. They may be subdivided roughly into B and T areas in which either B lymphocytes or T lymphocytes predominate (Parrott 1976). When selectively enriched populations of labelled B lymphocytes or T lymphocytes are injected intravenously they can be shown to migrate to specific B or T areas. Lymphocytes appear to migrate through the GALT by similar routes and processes, as occurs in other peripheral lymphatic tissue (Le-Fevre et al 1979).

Peyer's patches, located in the ileum of humans, consist of clusters of lymphoid follicles with well-defined structures. Recent studies have demonstrated that a specialized epithelial cell overlying Peyer's patches may facilitate the access of antigens to intestinal lymphoid tissues (Bochman & Cooper 1973, Pierce & Gowans 1975, Kagnoff 1977). Morphologically, these microfold cells (M cells), as they are called, have a paucity of microvilli, a poorly developed glycocalyx, and absence of lysosomal organelles. Horseradish peroxidase has been used by Owen & Jones (1974) and Owen (1977) to study antigen uptake by M cells. The marker is taken up into the specialized cells, rapidly released into the interstitial space, and processed by lymphoid cells circulating through the Peyer's patches. This mechanism of antigen transport in the gut appears to represent an important specialized access route for ingested antigen to reach lymphoid tissues and thereby stimulate the local and distant immune system. Not only do intact macromolecules appear to be processed by M cells, but also viruses (Wolf et al 1981) and bacteria (Inman 1983) which may be present in increased amounts in the malnourished individual. Indeed, as we shall discuss subsequently, there appears to be a significant increase in macromolecular transport across the intestine of malnourished animals.

The most studied mucosal defence mechanism of GALT is the synthesis and release of a special form of IgA, secretory IgA (SIgA), which is the predominant immunoglobulin of gastrointestinal secretions (Ogra 1970). Immunoglobulin A is produced by plasma cells in the lamina propria and passed into gut lumen after linkage to secretory piece in the epithelial cells (Walker 1976, Ogra 1979). Plasma cells that produce IgA reach the mucosa after a complicated migration of precursors initially stimulated in the distal ileum, via the specialized M cells. The antigens are in some way processed and lymphocytes sensitized and released, leading to the presence in the thoracic duct lymph of lymphocytes that stain for specific IgA antibody. Pierce & Gowans (1975) studied this migration using cholera toxin in rats in which antitoxin-containing cells were demonstrated in thoracic duct lymph following the intraduodenal presentation of toxin. They further reported that these lymphoid cells could eventually be found in the lamina propria, particularly at sites in which the antigen was first presented (Fig. 3.1). Pierce and his colleagues (Barry & Pierce 1979) have also showed, as we shall discuss later, a decrease in thoracic duct IgA containing lymphocytes in malnourished animals.

The major host defence mechanism of antibody of both SIgA (Heremans 1974, Walker 1978) and fragments of other Ig classes (Steele et al 1975) in the intestinal lumen is due to binding of antibody to antigen (immune exclusion), thereby preventing attachment to the epithelial surface. It has been suggested that IgA may also coat the intestinal epithelium and prevent bacterial adhesion to the epithelial surface, thereby suppressing the growth of certain bacterial pathogens (Williams & Gibbons 1972, Wright 1977, Rogers & Synge 1978). The quest for other potential activities of this immunoglobulin, such as opsonization and complement fixation, has been largely unsuccessful (Ottaway et al 1979).

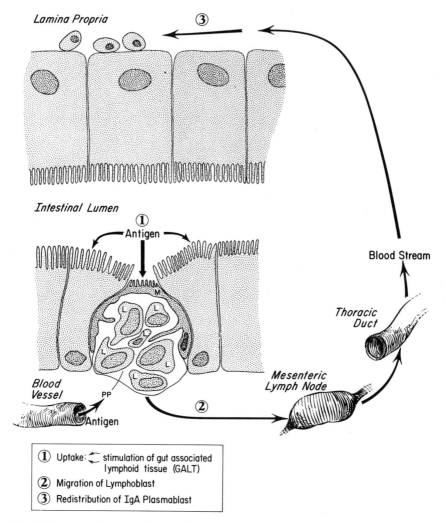

Lamina Propria

③

Intestinal Lumen

①
←Antigen→

Blood Stream

Thoracic Duct

Mesenteric Lymph Node

Blood Vessel
PP
Antigen

②

① Uptake: ⊃ stimulation of gut associated
              lymphoid tissue (GALT)
② Migration of Lymphoblast
③ Redistribution of IgA Plasmablast

Fig. 3.1 Diagram depicting a lymphoblast (or lymphocyte) in a Peyer's patch which is exposed to an antigen. The lymphoblast (or lymphocyte) is transported to a mesenteric lymph node and then to the thoracic duct. It enters the blood, by which it returns to the intestinal tract. In the lamina propria it further differentiates into an IgA plasma cell. (Reproduced with permission, Walker & Isselbacher 1977.)

Macrophages

Although macrophages of lung, peritoneal cavity, spleen, and liver have been discussed at length (Carr 1973), little published work has dealt directly with the origin, abundance, and activity of intestinal macrophages. Intestinal macrophages reside in the small intestine associated with GALT, surrounding the crypts of Lieberkuhn and in the villous core. Although these cells are similar to macrophages in other parts of the body, they lack several characteristics, including a specific nuclear and lysosomal morphologic appearance, phagocytic activity, lysosomal acid phosphatase, and membrane receptors for complement and the Fc portion of the IgG molecule (Carr & Wright 1978).

Macrophages carry out diverse functions in the intestinal tract, including phagocytosis, secretion, and participation in certain cell- and humoral-immune responses. Recent studies have shown that particulate matter absorbed and released by M cells in the Peyer's patch epithelium, reaches the subepithelial zone and is then engulfed by the macrophages of the region (Joel et al 1978, LeFevre et al 1978a, LeFevre et al 1978b).

CHANGES IN THE GASTROINTESTINAL IMMUNE SYSTEM WITH AGE

There is recent evidence to suggest that gastrointestinal immune function, and therefore intestinal host defences, are immature early in life (Walker 1976, Ogra 1979, Udall 1981). However, it has been noted that newborn infants ingesting breast milk may passively receive immune components that bottle-fed infants lack. In addition, recent studies indicate that breast milk may also stimulate the development of the intestinal immune defence (Pittard & Bill 1979a, 1979b). Additional studies of early feeding practices and intestinal and sytemic immunity indicate that the ingestion of a formula high in protein increases the synthesis and/or release of systemic immunoglobulins (Zoppi et al 1978, Zoppi et al 1982). Taken together, these studies provide evidence that early nutrition may modulate or influence intestinal immune development.

Humoral immunity

Bursa equivalent cells (B cells) present in GALT and scattered throughout the intestine are decreased in number in the intestine of newborns. Perkkio & Savilahti (1980) have noted a deficiency of immunoglobulin containing cells in the gut of human infants up to 12 days of age. Shortly after birth, intestinal IgM containing lymphocytes outnumber IgA cells (Allen & Porter 1977, Perkkio & Savilahti 1980). This is in contrast to later in life when IgA plasma cells are predominant.

There is also a reduction in salivary (Selner et al 1968), serum (Allansmith et al 1968) and stool (Haneberg & Aarskog 1975) IgA in newborns compared to older children and adults. Bùrgio et al (1980) measured secretory IgA in the saliva of healthy human subjects from two months to 27 years of age. He found a physiologic deficiency of SIgA during infancy and childhood and speculated that this deficiency may well play a role in the pathogenesis of infectious diseases of the respiratory and gastrointestinal tract frequent in this age group.

To evaluate the immune response in human infants Reiger and Rothberg

(1975) fed bovine serum albumin (BSA) to newborns delivered at different gestational ages and followed the development of serum anti-BSA-antibodies. Four of 5 infants 35 weeks gestation or older developed antibody to BSA whereas none of 8 infants younger than 35 weeks produced anti-BSA. However, factors other than gestational age appear to be important for a normal immune response. Studies have clearly demonstrated that newborn and germ-free animals exposed to a paucity of intestinal antigens have a striking absence of antibody-producing cells (Pollard & Sharon 1970, Ferguson & Parrott 1972). These observations emphasize the importance of age and local antigenic exposure of GALT in stimulating differentiation of lymphoid tissue capable of synthesizing antibodies at intestinal mucosal surfaces.

The observation that antigens present in the intestine stimulate the gastrointestinal immune system is important in view of the increased number of bacteria in the small intestine of individuals with PEM (Viteri & Schneider 1974, Gracey 1979). Bacterial overgrowth most certainly represents an increased antigen load to the immune system of the small bowel.

Cellular Immunity

Joel et al (1972) noted in mice an increase in cells migrating from the thymus to Peyer's patches very early in the neonatal period. Antigens may modify the traffic of T-lymphocytes into the epithelium the same way it influences cell traffic in the lamina propria (Reynolds 1980). With increasing age, the number of lymphocytes in the intestine increases markedly.

Macrophages

There are no studies which examine the function of macrophages and their role in the immune function of the intestine during development.

MALNUTRITION AND GASTROINTESTINAL IMMUNE FUNCTION

Patients with kwashiorkor tend to have the severe intestinal morphologic changes, the greatest disruption of gastrointestinal function, and most probably the greatest impairment of gastrointestinal immunity. In contrast to this, patients with marasmus in many instances have what appears to be a normal intestine with minimal dysfunction (Walker 1980).

The effects of both types of malnutrition on gastrointestinal immunity has been studied in animals and humans. But the studies have focused for the most part on humoral and not cellular immunity. Although there is a considerable amount of data supporting the concept that the systemic cellular immune system is affected dramatically in the malnourished host, very little is known about cellular immune function in the gastrointestinal tract of malnourished individuals.

Humoral immunity

Bursa equivalent (B) cells that differentiate into IgA producing plasma cells in the small intestine have been studied in underfed newborn mice (Wade et al 1982). Wade and associates (1982) allowed female mice to nurture litters of 4, 9 or 20 pups. This produced a state of obesity (litters of 4) or protein-energy malnutrition (litters of 20). Litters of 9 were considered controls. Overfeeding (litters of 4) during the suckling period did not change the development and the number of IgA plasma cells in the small intestine. In contrast, the weanling protein-energy malnourished mice (litters of 20) had shorter intestines, reduced weight of the gut mucosa and reduced villous length. Protein-energy malnutrition limited only to the suckling period, had no marked effect on the development of IgA intestinal plasma cells, however a diminished number of these cells was observed when a more severe and prolonged malnourished state was induced (Wade et al 1982).

Barry & Pierce (1979) observed more dramatic effects of malnutrition on intestinal immunity. These investigators assessed the effect of protein deprivation on the gastrointestinal immune response to cholera toxoid/toxin in 7-week-old rats. Diets of control and protein-deficient animals differed only in protein content, containing 24 per cent and 3.2 per cent protein respectively. After 6 weeks of feeding, control animals weighed 240 g and protein-deficient animals weighed 125 g. The investigators then quantitated the number of large thoracic duct lymphocytes (TDL) and TDL containing IgA. There were diminished numbers of large TDL in the protein deprived animals suggesting an impaired mucosal immune response to enteric antigens during malnutrition (Table 3.1). This was confirmed by determining the number of specific antitoxin containing cells in rats immunized orally with cholera toxoid/toxin. Compared to protein-deprived animals, rats fed the control diet showed an increased number of antitoxin-containing lympholasts after an oral dose of toxoid/toxin followed by a booster dose of toxoid (Fig. 3.2). The authors found that this impairment of mucosal immune

Table 3.1   Thoracic duct lymphocytes (TDL) in unimmunized normal and protein-deficient rats (geometric mean of cells per hour $\times 10^{-6} \pm$ s.e.mean)

Type	Total TDL	Large TDL	TDL containing IgA
Normal diet	21 (1.1)	2.1 (1.2)	0.24 (1.3)
Low-protein diet	9.0 (1.1)	0.61 (1.1)	0.13 (1.2)
P	< 0.001	< 0.001	0.06

Reproduced with permission (Barry & Pierce 1979).

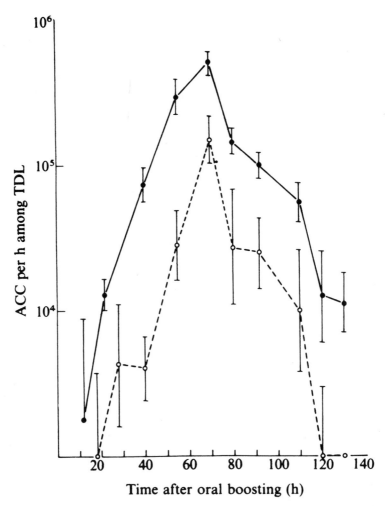

Fig. 3.2 Antitoxin-containing cells (ACC) among thoracic duct lymph from normal (●) and protein-deficient (○) rats after oral immunization with CT. The priming dose was crude toxoid and crude toxin given at age 11 weeks. The booster dose was crude toxoid given 2 weeks later. The thoracic duct was cannulated and antitoxin-containing cells among TDL were counted using a fluorescent antibody technique specific for cholera antitoxin. (Reproduced with permission, Barry & Pierce 1979.)

response to cholera toxoid/toxin was rapidly reversed by refeeding (Barry & Pierce 1979).

Studies in humans have also documented changes in the humoral component of the intestinal immune system in malnourished children. Sirisinha and colleagues (1975) measured the concentration of total protein, IgG, IgA and albumin in the nasopharyngeal washings of children with PEM. The investigators studied 24 children with PEM who were 1 to 5 years of age and 23 similarly aged normal children. The PEM children were classified as having kwashiorkor, marasmus, or marasmus-kwashiorkor according to clinical criteria. Some subjects had vitamin A deficiency and two thirds of the malnourished group had infections. It was noted that only secretory IgA (SIgA) concentrations in the nasopharyngeal wash were significantly lower in the PEM compared to normal children. Other proteins were not significantly affected (IgG and albumin). The decreased SIgA levels remained significantly lower than control values through hospital day 70 before returning to normal (Sirisinha et al 1975).

Chandra (1975) assessed mucosal immune response in malnourished and well-nourished children. In his study, 20 boys, aged 1–4 years, were classified as malnourished on the basis of a history of reduced dietary intake, loss of subcutaneous tissue and hair changes. Weight and height were 50–70 per cent of the mean on reference growth charts. Twenty age- and sex-matched healthy children served as controls. A single dose of live attenuated polio virus vaccine was given by mouth to 10 seronegative children in each group. Another 10 malnourished patients and 10 healthy controls received one dose of live attenuated measles vaccine. Serum and nasopharyngeal secretions were obtained each week the first month after immunization and thereafter every two weeks for one to two months. Secretory IgA concentrations in nasal washings and serum neutralizing antibody titres to poliovirus type 1 and measles were quantitated. Immunoglobulin A was significantly reduced in the nasopharyngeal secretions of malnourished patients. Seroconversion after poliovirus vaccine was achieved in 8 of the 10 malnourished children and in all the healthy controls. Specific IgA antibody titres to poliovirus in nasopharyngeal washings (Fig. 3.3) were significantly lower in the malnourished children compared to controls ($p < 0.01$). The amount of nasopharyngeal measles neutralizing antibody titre at all test periods after immunization was also significantly lower in those with malnutrition ($p < 0.01$). Chandra (1975) postulated that impaired secretory antibody response in malnourished children may contribute to viral and bacterial infections and predispose malnourished children to life-threatening complications.

Reddy and collaborators (1976) studied the secretory IgA system of 38 malnourished children between 1 and 6 years of age. The children were divided into 3 groups on the basis of weight for age. Twelve children whose weights were above 80 per cent of the standard (Indian Council of Medical Research 1972) were considered normal, while 10 children whose values were between 60–80 per cent of the standard but who had no clinical signs of malnutrition were classified as mild-moderate PEM. Sixteen children with weights below 60 per cent of the standard were considered to be suffering from severe PEM (10 of these children had signs of kwashiorkor and the other 6 were marasmic). Sixteen of the 38 children had diarrhoea. Blood samples were obtained from all the subjects for estimation of serum immunoglobulin and albumin levels. Duodenal fluid, saliva, tears and nasal secretions were also collected for IgA determination. The results of the study indicate that in children suffering from kwashiorkor and marasmus

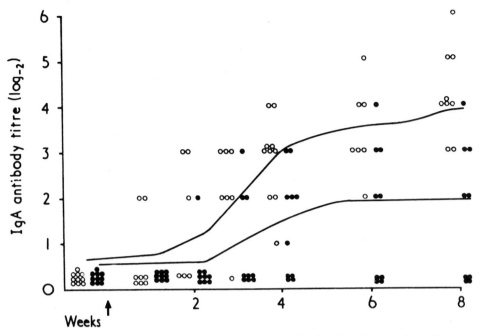

Fig. 3.3 Level of specific IgA antibody to poliovirus type I in healthy (○) and malnourished (•) children before and after a single oral dose of live attenuated trivalent poliovirus vaccine. (Reproduced with permission, Chandra 1975.)

(severe PEM) the concentration of IgA in duodenal fluid, saliva, nasal secretions, and tears was significantly reduced but returned to normal after four weeks of adequate nutrition. The concentration of secretory IgA in these body fluids was not different when samples obtained from children with mild to moderate PEM was compared to those from normal children (Reddy et al 1976).

More recently, Green & Heyworth (1980) extended the findings of these earlier studies. They obtained jejunal biopsies from 20 well-nourished children (average age 12.8 months) with gastroenteritis, and 20 children with protein-energy malnutrition (average age 20 months). The 20 children with PEM were classified as having marasmus, kwashiorkor or marasmus-kwashiorkor. Intestinal biopsy specimens were examined by immunofluorescent techniques for lymphocytes containing immunoglobulins A, G, M, E, and D. Compared with previous studies of normal infants, the children with gastroenteritis showed a moderate increase in IgA-containing cells, a large increase in IgM-containing cells, and no change in IgG-containing cells. In contrast there was a pronounced and highly significant decrease in IgA-containing cells in the jejunal mucosa of the children with protein-energy malnutrition. No significant differences were noted between the populations of IgG-, IgM, IgE- and IgD-containing cells in the two groups (Green & Heyworth 1980).

Each of the above studies support the hypothesis that the increased incidence of intestinal mucosal infection in malnourished children may result from defective antibody production. However, not all studies are in agreement with this point (Barry & Pierce 1979). Bell, Gracey and their collaborators (Bell et al, 1976) did not find a deficiency of intestinal IgA in malnourished patients. These investigators obtained duodenal fluid samples and quantitated intestinal immunoglobulin levels in undernourished Indonesian children with enteric infections and normally nourished Indonesians with and without enteric infections. Immunoglobulin levels were also determined in duodenal samples from Australian Aboriginal children suffering undernutrition and normal Caucasian children. The investigators found that children with enteric infections had elevated levels of intestinal immunoglobulins irrespective of their nutritional status. Intestinal infections increased IgG concentrations more than secretory IgA in the age groups examined. However, it appeared likely that some of the IgG was serum-derived whereas the IgA most likely was locally produced. The investigators concluded that there was no apparent deficiency in the capacity of undernourished children to manufacture and secrete immunoglobulin in the gut. Although, this study appears to contradict the results obtained by others, several points should be emphasized. As noted earlier, it is difficult to separate the effect of malnutrition from that of infection. Malnutrition may depress immune function as Barry & Pierce (1979) demonstrated in animals and Chandra (1975) showed in humans and intestinal infection may stimulate immune function as Green and Heyworth (1980) noted. When both malnutrition and infection are present, it is difficult to assess which is the more important. Secondly, acute gastroenteritis may cause a protein-losing enteropathy which increases IgG concentrations in intestinal secretions (Dossetor & Whittle 1975). The loss of serum (Ig(s) into the intestine in acute gastroenteritis is not related to suppression or stimulation of the immune system.

Cellular immunity

The effect of a low protein diet on antibody-dependent cell-mediated cytotoxicity (ADCC) and IgA concentrations in the intestine of different aged mice was assessed by Lim et al (1981). Both ADCC activity and intestinal IgA concentration in mice were shown to reach mature levels at 17 weeks of age. Lim and his coworkers found that a low protein diet had a greater suppressive effect on IgA concentration than on cell-mediated cytotoxicity. The depression of intestinal IgA was directly related to the chronicity of the low protein diet. Short-term exposure to the low-protein diet (8 weeks) did not affect dramatically ADCC activity and IgA concentration.

It is well known that in PEM there is a generalized decrease in mature circulating T lymphocytes, although there is a relative increase in lymphyocytes free of identifying markers, so-called null cells (Chandra 1977). However, no human studies of intestinal T cells or null cells have been performed in subjects with protein-energy malnutrition.

Phagocytosis

Malnourished monkeys and rodents have a depression of uptake of colloidal carbon and *Escherichia coli* by the fixed (tissue) mononuclear cell system (Keusch 1982). Studies in mice, which have confirmed the depression of phagocytosis by the fixed mononuclear cells in protein deficient animals, have also demonstrated that this decrease was proportional to the reduction in the sizes of liver and spleen (Keusch 1982). No studies of phagocytosis has been conducted using cells obtained from the intestinal tract of malnourished animals or humans.

Complement

With the exception of C4, there is a decrease in the concentration of all components of the classical pathway of complement activation in PEM. There is also a significant impairment of haemolytic complement activity (Ch_{50}) as measured with sensitized sheep erythrocytes (Keusch 1982). To date, no studies of the complement system function in the intestinal tract have been performed in malnourished animals or humans.

GASTROINTESTINAL BARRIER DEFENCE DURING MALNUTRITION

It has been suggested that a general disruption of the mucosal barrier occurs during PEM and that potentially dangerous antigens may gain access to the host (Walker 1980). An increase in macromolecular transport across the intestine during protein calorie malnutrition has been documented in animals. Worthington and colleagues (1974a, 1974b, 1976) have shown that severely and chronically protein-malnourished rats have an increased uptake of intact protein into intestinal epithelial cells. Their data have been confirmed in our laboratory by Dr Deborah Rothman (1982a, 1982b) who has shown that radiolabelled bovine serum albumin (BSA) is transported across the intestinal barrier and into blood in increased quantities in animals which are severely and chronically protein-energy malnourished.

Dr Rothman (Rothman et al 1983) has also recently assessed macromolecular transport in animals during short-term malnutrition. She starved newborn rabbits for 72 hours immediately following birth. Thereafter, a dose of BSA proportional to body weight was given to control and experimental animals. Four hours later blood was obtained by cardiac puncture and plasma analysed for immunoreactive BSA (iBSA) compared to controls (16.8 μg/ml). She has found that animals starved from birth had increased plasma i-BSA (22.7 μg/ml). The permeability of the small intestine was also evaluated in animals allowed to nurse for 5 or 14 days of life and then starved for 72 hours. There was no difference in the quantity of i-BSA recovered from the plasma in the older starved groups compared to age-matched controls. Her studies suggest that barrier function of the intestine is altered more drastically by the effects of PEM in the immediate neonatal period than later in infancy.

SUMMARY

Studies that have examined the effect of malnutrition on gastrointestinal immunity suggest that at least the humoral arm of the immune system is impaired in protein-energy malnutrition. However, nutritional status has not been completely and stringently controlled in many human studies, and many malnourished children studied have been infected. Therefore, additional, better controlled studies are necessary. In addition, much has yet to be learned concerning intestinal cell-mediated immune function during malnutrition. Hopefully, investigators will accept the challenge to investigate this important area and develop new insights which may enable us to better care for malnourished children.

REFERENCES

Allansmith M, McClellan B H, Butterworth M, Maloney J R 1968 The development of immunoglobulin levels in man. Journal of Pediatrics 72: 276–290

Allen W D, Porter P 1977 The relative frequencies and distribution of immunoglobulin-bearing cells in the intestinal mucosa of neonatal and weaned pigs and their significance in the development of secretory immunity. Immunology 32: 819–824

Barry W S, Pierce N F 1979 Protein deprivation causes reversible impairment of mucosal immune response to cholera toxoid/toxin in rat gut. Nature 281: 64–65

Bell R G, Turner K J, Gracey M, Suharjono, Sunoto 1976 Serum and small intestinal immunoglobulin levels in undernourished children. The American Journal of Clinical Nutrition 29: 392–397

Bockman D E, Cooper M D 1973 Pinocytosis by epithelium associated with lymphoid follicles in the bursa of Fabricius, appendix and Peyer's patches. An electron microscopic study. American Journal of Anatomy 136: 455–477

Burgio G R, Lanzavecchia A, Plebani A, Jayakar S, Ugazio A G 1980 Ontogeny of secretory immunity: levels of secretory IgA and natural antibodies in saliva. Pediatric Research 14: 1111–1114

Carr I 1973 The fixed macrophage. In: The macrophage, a review of ultrastructure and function. Academic Press, London, p 20–40

Carr I, Wright J 1978 The reticuloendothelial and mononuclear phagocyte systems and the macrophage. Canadian Medical Association Journal 118: 882–891

Chandra R K 1975 Reduced secretory antibody response to live attenuated measles and poliovirus vaccines in malnourished children. British Medical Journal ii: 583–585

Chandra R K 1977 Lymphocyte subpopulations in human malnutrition: cytotoxic and suppressor cells. Pediatrics 59: 423–427

Dossetor J F B, Whittle H C 1975 Protein-losing enteropathy and malabsorption in acute measles enteritis. British Medical Journal ii: 592–593

Ferguson A, Parrott D M V 1972 The effect of antigen deprivation on thymus-dependent and thymus-independent lymphocytes in the small intestine of the mouse. Clinical and Experimental Immunology 12: 477–488

Gomez F, Galvan R R, Cravioto J, Frenk S 1955 Malnutrition in infancy and childhood, with special reference to kwashiorkor. Advances in Pediatrics 7: 131–169

Gracey M 1979 The contaminated small bowel syndrome: Pathogenesis, diagnosis, and treatment. The American Journal of Clinical Nutrition 32: 234–243

Green F, Heyworth B 1980 Immunoglobulin-containing cells in jejunal mucosa of children with protein-energy malnutrition and gastroenteritis. Archives of Disease in Childhood 55: 380–383

Haneberg B, Aarskog D 1975 Human immunoglobulins in healthy infants and children and in some diseases affecting the intestinal tract or the immune system. Clinical and Experimental Immunology 22: 210–222

Heremans J F 1974 Immunoglobulin A. In: Sela M (ed) The antigens, vol 2. Academic Press, New York, p 365–522

Indian Council of Medical Research 1972 Growth and physical development of Indian infants and children. Technical Report Series No. 18, p 24

Inman L R, Cantey J R 1983 Specific adherence of Escherichia coli (strain RDEC-1) to membranous (M) cells of the Peyer's patch in Escherichia coli diarrhea in the rabbit. The Journal of Clinical Investigation 71: 1–8

Joel D D, Hess M W, Cottier H 1972 Magnitude and pattern of thymic lymphocyte migration in neonatal mice. Journal of Experimental Medicine 135: 907–923

Joel D D, Laissue J A, Le Fevre M E 1978 Distribution and fate of ingested carbon particles in mice. Journal of the Reticuloendothelial Society 24: 477–487

Kagnoff M F 1977 Functional characteristics of Peyer's patch lymphoid cells. IV. Effect of antigen feeding on the frequency of antigen-specific B cells. Journal of Immunology 118: 992–997

Keusch G T 1982 Immune function in the malnourished host. Pediatric Annals 11; 12: 1004–1014

Le Fevre M E, Olivo R, Joel D D 1978a Accumulation of latex particles in Peyer's patches and their subsequent appearance in villi and mesenteric lymph nodes. Proceedings of the Society for Experimental Biology and Medicine. 159: 298–302

Le Fevre M E,Vanderhoff J W, Laissue J A, Joel D D 1978b Accumulation of 2-μm latex particles in mouse Peyer's patches during chronic latex feeding. Experientia 34: 120–122

Le Fevre M E, Hammer R, Joel D D 1979 Macrophages of the mammalian small intestine: A review. Journal of Reticuloendothelial Society 26: 553–573

Lim T S, Messiha N, Watson R R 1981 Immune components of the intestinal mucosa of aging and protein-deficient mice. Immunology 43: 401–407

Merritt R J, Suskind R M 1979 Nutritional survey of hospitalized pediatric patients. American Journal of Clinical Nutrition 32: 1320–1325

Ogra P L 1979 Ontogeny of the local immune system. Pediatrics 64: 765–774

Ottaway C A, Rose M L, Parrott D M V 1979 The gut as an immunological system. In: Crane R K (ed) Gastrointestinal physiology 3. International Review of Physiology, vol 19. University Park Press, Baltimore, p 323–356

Owen R L 1977 Sequential uptake of horseradish peroxidase by lymphoid follicle epithelium of Peyer's patches in the normal unobstructed mouse intestine: an ultrastructure study. Gastroenterology 72: 440–451

Owen R L, Jones A L 1974 Epithelial cell specialization within human Peyer's patches: an ultrastructural study of intestinal lymphoid follicles. Gastroenterology 66: 189–203

Parrott D M V 1976 The gut as a lymphoid organ. Clinical Gastroenterology 5: 211–228

Perkkio M, Savilahti E 1980 Time of appearance of immunoglobulin-containing cells in the mucosa of the neonatal intestine. Pediatric Research 14: 953–955

Pierce N F, Gowans J L 1975 Cellular kinetics of the intestinal immune response to cholera toxoid in rats. Journal of Experimental Medicine 142: 1550–1563

Pittard W B III, Bill K 1979a Differentiation of cord blood lymphocytes into IgA-producing cells in response to breast milk stimulatory factor. Clinical Immunology and Immunopathology 13: 430–434

Pittard W B III, Bill K 1979b Immunoregulation of breast milk cells. Cellular Immunology 42: 437–441

Pollard M, Sharon N 1970 Responses of Peyer's patches in germ-free mice to antigenic stimulation. Infection and Immunity 2: 96–100

Reddy V, Raghuramulu N, Bhaskaram C 1976 Secretory IgA in protein-calorie malnutrition. Archives of Disease in Childhood 51: 871–874

Reiger C H, Rothberg R M 1975 Development of the capacity to produce specific antibody to an ingested food antigen in the premature infant. Journal of Pediatrics 87: 515–518

Reynolds J 1980 Gut-associated lymphoid tissue in lamb before and after birth. Monographs in Allergy 16: 187–202

Rogers H J, Synge C 1978 Bacteriostatic effect of human milk on E. coli. The role of IgA. Immunology 34: 19–28

Rothman D, Latham M C, Walker W A 1982a Transport of macromolecules in malnourished animals. I Evidence for increased uptake of intestinal antigens. Nutrition Research 2: 467–473

Rothman D, Latham M C, Walker W A 1982b Transport of macromolecules in malnourished animals. II Intravenous clearance after antigen absorption. Nutrition Research 2: 475–480

Rothman D, Udall J, Pang K, Walker W A 1983 The effect of short-term starvation on mucosal barrier function in the newborn rabbit. Pediatric Research 17: 199A

Scrimshaw N S 1975 Interactions of malnutrition and infection: Advances in understanding. In: Olson R E (ed), Protein-calorie malnutrition. Academic Press, New York, p 353–367

Selner J C, Merrill D A, Claman H N 1968 Salivary immunoglobulins and albumin: development during the newborn period. Journal of Pediatrics 72: 685–689

Sirisinha S, Suskind R, Edelman R, Asvapaka C, Olson R E 1975 Secretory and serum IgA in children with protein-calorie malnutrition. Pediatrics 55: 166–170

Steele E J, Chaicumpa W, Rowley D 1975 Further evidence for cross-linking as a protective factor in experimental cholera: properties of antibody fragment. Journal of Infectious Diseases 132: 175–180

Suskind R M 1975 Gastrointestinal changes in the malnourished child. Pediatric Clinics of North America 22: 873–883

Udall J N 1981 Maturation of intestinal host defense: an update. Nutrition Research 1: 399–418

Udall J N, Walker W A 1983 Immunological function of the developing gut. In: Warshaw J B (ed) The biological basis of reproductive and developmental medicine. Elsevier Biomedical, New York, p 221–238

Viteri F E 1981 Primary protein-energy malnutrition: clinical, biochemical, and metabolic changes. In: Suskind R M (ed) Textbook of pediatric nutrition. Raven Press, New York, p 189–215

Viteri F E, Schneider R E 1974 Gastrointestinal alterations in protein-calorie malnutrition. Medical Clinics of North American 58: 1487–1505

Wade S, Lemonnier D, Alexiu A, Bocquet L 1982 Effect of early postnatal under- and overnutrition on the development of IgA plasma cells in mouse gut. Journal of Nutrition 112: 1047–1051

Walker W A 1976 Host defense mechanisms in the gastrointestinal tract. Pediatrics 57: 901–916

Walker W A 1978 Antigen handling by the gut. Archives of Diseases in Childhood 53: 527–531

Walker W A 1980 Cellular and immune changes in the gastrointestinal tract in malnutrition. In: Winik M (ed) Nutrition and gastroenterology. John Wiley & Sons, New York, ch 14, p 197–218

Walker W A, Isselbacher K J 1977 Intestinal antibodies. New England Journal of Medicine 297: 767–773

Waterlow J C 1972 Classification and definition of protein-calorie malnutrition. British Medical Journal 3: 566–569

Waterlow J C 1973 Note on the assessment and classification of protein-energy malnutrition in children. Lancet ii: 87–89

Williams R C, Gibbons R J 1972 Inhibition of bacterial adherence by secretory immunoglobulin A: a mechanism of antigen disposal. Science 1977: 697–699

Wolf J L, Rubin D H, Finberg R, Kauffman R S, Sharpe A H, Trier J S, et al 1981 Intestinal M cells: a pathway for entry of reovirus into the host. Science 212: 471–472

Worthington B S, Boatman E S 1974a The influence of protein malnutrition on ileal permeability to macromolecules in the rat. American Journal of Digestive Disease 19: 43–55

Worthington B S, Boatman E S, Kenny G E 1974b Intestinal absorption of intact proteins in normal and protein-deficient rats. American Journal of Clincal Nutrition 27: 276–286

Worthington B S, Syrotuck J 1976 Intestinal permeability to large particles in normal and protein deficient adult rats. Journal of Nutrition 106: 20–32

Wright R 1977 Normal immune responses in the gut and immunodeficiency disorders. In: Tuck J (ed) Immunology of gastrointestinal and liver disease. Edward Arnold Publishers, London, p 1–15

Zee P, Walters T, Mitchell C 1970 Nutrition and poverty in preschool children. A nutritional survey of preschool children from impoverished black families, Memphis. Journal of the American Medical Association 213: 739–742

Zoppi G, Zamboni G, Siviero M, Bellini P, Cancellieri M L 1978 Gamma-globulin level and dietary protein intake during the first year of life. Pediatrics 62: 1010–1018

Zoppi G, Gerosa F, Pezzini A, Bassani N, Rizzotti P, Bellini P, et al 1982 Immunocompetence and dietary protein intake in early infancy. Journal of Pediatric Gastroenterology and Nutrition 1: 175–182

In the context of this chapter it would be helpful to be able to ascribe priorities in terms of the strength of the associations of various diarrhoeal agents with malnutrition. If we accept that catabolism is not a major feature of diarrhoeal disease then two aspects of the nutrition–infection interaction emerge as important, namely impaired nutrient intake and nutrient losses in the stool (see Fig. 4.1), the latter usually being related to nutrient malabsorption.

Some degree of anorexia is common in cases of diarrhoea, as in many other infections, and nutrient intake may be further compromised by vomiting or even withholding of food. A drastic fall in intake of weaning foods has been documented in children with diarrhoea in a number of community studies and has been confirmed also in hospital studies. Molla and colleagues (1983) showed that in hospitalized children with non-invasive diarrhoea of bacterial origin, if food was made available, the period of anorexia lasted for about four days but this was often followed by a period of enhanced appetite. The picture was rather different in the case of rotavirus, when lower intakes were observed for more prolonged periods. In the hospital situation again, Hoyle et al (1980) showed loss of appetite to be selective, with breast milk intake being much less affected than that of solids or semi-solids.

Malabsorption of various nutrients in the acute stages of diarrhoea varied considerably with the aetiological agent causing the illness. By two weeks post-recovery, however, the absorption of calories had improved to between 80 and 90 per cent irrespective of the aetiology of the diarrhoea (Molla et al 1984). In fact it has been known for some time (Chung 1948) that even though increasing nutrient intakes in cases of diarrhoea lead to increased stool losses, the net retention is improved. More surprising are the results of a study in Bangladesh where relationships between nutrient intakes and stool losses were studied with respect to nutritional status of the subjects (Molla et al 1984). These workers concluded that in the absence of severe mucosal damage, as in shigellosis, children with severe malnutrition tended to eat more and absorb more than their better nourished counterparts.

The above findings relate largely to patients hospitalized on account of acute dehydrating gastroenteritis. They tend to be supported by the results of longitudinal community studies in rural Bangladesh (Black et al 1983) with respect to *Shigella* but not necessarily other diarrhoeal agents. There enterotoxigenic *E. coli* diarrhoeas were found to have a significant negative effect on bimonthly weight gain, whilst shigelloses had a similar effect on bimonthly and annual linear growth increments. The incidence rate of shigellosis was only half that of ETEC diarrhoea but the duration of attacks were longer. Diarrhoeal attacks of indeterminate origin showed a non-significant negative association with growth in both height and weight which was greatest in those attacks of long duration (> 10 days). The relative lack of impact of rotavirus gastroenteritis on growth may well have been due to the infrequency with which prolonged attacks occurred, though is more difficult to explain in the light of the findings described in the above hospital series in respect of intake and absorptive function.

Nevertheless the bulk of the evidence points to the benefit of minimizing periods of food withdrawal and of attempting to restore children to a good nutrient intake as early as possible in the recovery stage of diarrhoea. Though some increase in stool losses may be observed in these circumstances the old maxim, 'the child is more important than the stool' (Park 1924) is still a good one. These points will be considered in more detail in Chapters 10 and 11 dealing with the treatment of diarrhoea.

To turn to the preventive aspects of diarrhoeal disease and malnutrition, it has been stated (Mata et al 1976, Rowland et al 1977, Black et al 1983) that health and more particularly growth in early childhood could be markedly improved, if not normalized, by the elimination of diarrhoeal illnesses and there is no doubt that this is a highly desirable, if currently impractical, goal. Prevention of diarrhoeal illness will be discussed in a later chapter; the nature of the strategies involved is determined by epidemiological aspects of the transmission of diarrhoea and also by the nature of its association with malnutrition. This synergistic relationship is one of the best documented examples of the nutrition–infection interaction and is illustrated in its simplest form in Figure 4.1, with some basic mechanisms which are commonly invoked. Of course, statistical associations do not prove cause and effect but in at least one of the major longitudinal studies referred to above it has been argued that diarrhoea is a major cause of impairment of growth, (Rowland et al 1977) a view which is widely held. Equally common is the entirely compatible concept of malnutrition in some way predisposing towards diarrhoeal disease and enhancing its severity. There is relatively little good data to support this. What there is shows that diarrhoeal duration (Palmer et al 1976, Martinez & Chavez 1979) and perhaps incidence is increased in malnourished children. Severity may also be increased within this group as judged by weight loss (Mata et al 1977) and perhaps stool losses but this last issue is not yet fully resolved. One intervention study which purported to show that the provision of a food supplement to children reduced the

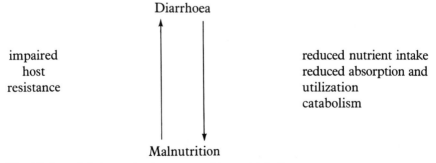

Fig. 4.1 Synergistic interaction between nutrition and infection

diarrhoeal morbidity (Wray 1978) has been received with considerable reservations (Rosenberg 1978).

CONTAMINATED FOOD AND WATER

Returning to more conventional aspects of epidemiology, gastroenteritis caused by bacterial pathogens is without exception believed to be spread by the faecal-oral route, i.e. the passage of faecal material from an infected person to the alimentary tract of another subject. In endemic situations, particularly where young children are concerned, a detailed knowledge of this route of transmission rarely exists. Clearly the normal developmental behaviour of older infants and toddlers actively exploring their surroundings at ground level, instinctively transferring objects from hand to mouth in an environment where they and others, even animals, have often been allowed to defaecate indiscriminately, predisposes strongly to the acquisition of faecal pathogens. This is not an easy risk to quantify. There have been a number of studies, however, of selected aspects of environmental hygiene relating to food and water contamination which offer circumstantial evidence of potentially important routes of transmission of bacterial pathogens.

In The Gambia, rural village well water supplies were shown to be faecally contaminated with material both of human and animal origin (Fig. 4.2).

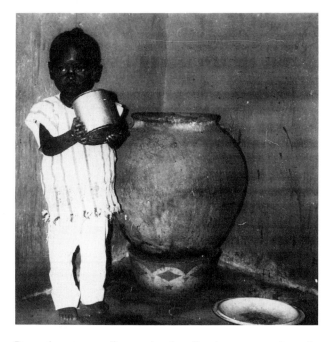

Fig. 4.2a–c Domestic water supplies are already polluted at source and may become further contaminated before consumption. (Courtesy Dr R G Whitehead)

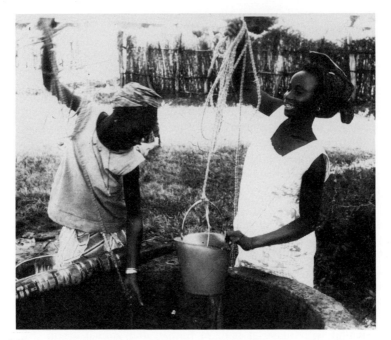

Fig. 4.2b

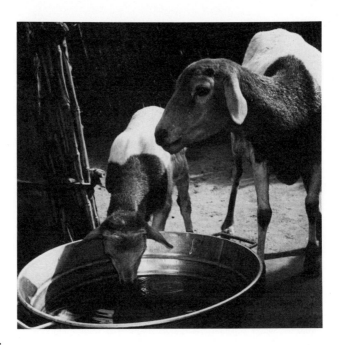

Fig. 4.2c

Pollution increased 10- to 100-fold within days of the onset of the rains and persisted at these higher levels throughout the rainy season, which was also the period of highest diarrhoeal prevalence (Barrell & Rowland 1979a). Food contamination showed similar seasonal variation, the worst examples being documented in early weaning foods in which there was a delay of some hours between preparation and consumption, thus providing the opportunity for bacterial replication and overgrowth. In addition to the presence of faecal markers, gut pathogens were also identified, many of which were known to be associated with food poisoning as well as acute gastroenteritis (Barrell & Rowland 1979b).

Detailed studies of the process of domestic food preparation in a Gambian village demonstrated a multiplicity of points at which contaminants might enter and indicated the importance of the contribution of polluted water to the picture (Barrell & Rowland 1980). Some of these points are illustrated in Figures 4.2 and 4.3 and indicated schematically in Table 4.3. It may be seen from this representation, that opportunities for contamination of weaning foods by one or more agents occur at every stage of preparation and it is instructive to consider these problems individually:

1. *Bacillus cereus* would appear to be an almost inevitable hazard associated with cereals. It occurs in 70 per cent of uncooked rice samples in the United Kingdom. It may unquestionably give rise to food poisoning epidemics through inadequately cooked and, particularly, reheated rice dishes but to what extent it contributes to childhood diarrhoeas in LDCs is not known.

2. *Polluted well water* could be eliminated from the process of domestic flour production by the use of a hand grinder which obviates the need for wetting the grain. Water used in the actual food preparation should, of course, be thoroughly boiled first but constraints imposed by time, heating and storage facilities combine to make this simple routine an arduous imposition for already overworked women.

3. *Gross contamination of the environment*, of which roaming livestock are the most easily remedied cause, should be controllable with care, but a leaky hut with mud floors is almost impossible to keep clean in the rainy season and the problem of general hygiene in the more squalid and poverty-stricken environments is almost insoluble.

4. *The residual contamination of washed utensils* is particularly heavy in the case of traditional calabashes. It may largely be eliminated by the use of intact metal pots and a cleaning agent such as soap. The problem of the polluted water in which they are washed may be overcome by careful drying in an uncontaminated area if such is available.

5. *Personal hygiene.* There is no doubt that the young infant of four months who requires some diet in addition to breast milk is highly vulnerable. Disciplined personal hygiene and the standard of food handling by the mother is all-important in this respect, whether using traditional or imported weaning foods, and again the relevance of clean accessible water supplies is obvious.

Fig. 4.3a–f Contamination of food, which may not always be readily avoidable, occurs at virtually every stage of preparation (see text for further details). (Courtesy Dr R G Whitehead)

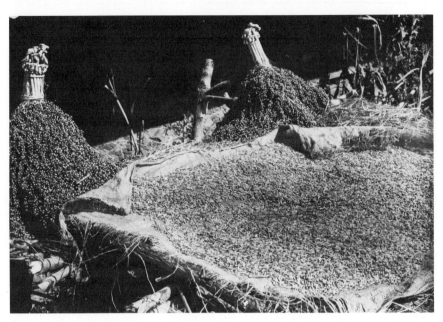

a

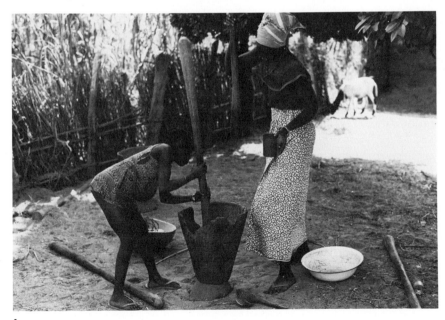

b

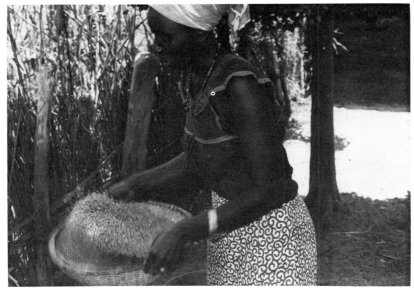

c

d

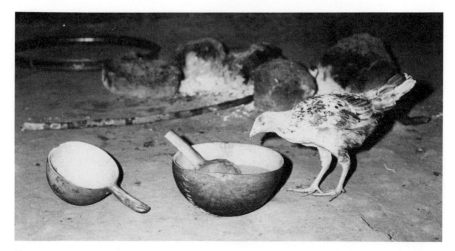

e

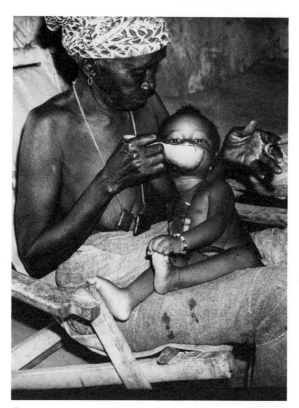

f

Table 4.3 Aspects of traditional Gambian weaning food preparation and hygiene related to opportunities for contamination

Water	Drawn from well Transported and stored in hut Fig. 4.2a, b, c	— all surface water faecally contamination — levels of contamination tend to fall on storage but fresh contaminants may be introduced by dipping into main container.
Stored grain	Fig. 4.3a	— *Bacillus cereus* ubiquitous[1]
Preparation	Pounding in pestle and mortar Fig. 4.3b Winnowing after sun-drying Fig. 4.3c Flour mixed with cold water	— damped with polluted well water[2] — may be contaminated by fomites or passing livestock[3] — utensils retain residual contaminants[4] after washing in well water — more organisms from admixed well water[2] — faecal and other organisms introduced by the food handlers[5]
Cooking	Gruel heated but not boiled Fig. 4.3c	— *B. cereus* spores and even some faecal organisms are not destroyed during cooking[6]
Interval before cooking	Some food may be eaten as soon as cool[6] Remaining food is set aside and eaten	— may be further contaminated by livestock[3] and fomites[4] Fig. 4.3e — rapid bacterial proliferation occurs in high ambient temperatures[7] Fig. 4.3f

1–7 See text for explanatory notes

6. *Cooking.* Contrary to popular belief, the process of cooking does not eliminate all the contamination that precedes it (Barrell & Rowland 1980). Sustained boiling produces a food which is too glutinous for the young infant to consume. It is not generally practised and, though numbers of bacteria fall during cooking, organisms are not eliminated. Time and inadequate cooking/heating facilities may be additional constraints at this point. Fortunately, foods for older children such as steamed foods and multimixes, though still contaminated to an unacceptable degree, are more satisfactorily treated by the normal cooking process.

7. *The problem of bacterial multiplication in food* after cooking is the most important single aspect of food handling. It applies to solid food as well as gruels and milk. Even minor degrees of contamination in freshly prepared food may give rise to massive levels after only a few hours at the ambient temperatures which prevail in many LDCs. Whether or not any one meal contains an infecting dose of a diarrhoeal pathogen, the repeated consumption by the child of subinfective doses in heavily contaminated food may be

one contributory cause to the weanling diarrhoea syndrome (Gordon et al 1963) which will be referred to below.

Though this particular scenario is derived specifically from studies in The Gambia, there is no doubt that it is of broader relevance where infant weaning foods are prepared in unhygienic settings in rural areas and in urban slums. These studies provide circumstantial evidence indicating the potential importance of domestic water and weaning food contamination in the transmission of gut pathogens. Subsequent studies in Bangladesh by Black et al (1981) have indicated relationships of a more precise nature. For example, contaminated domestic water supplies were found to be an important source of enterotoxigenic *E. coli* in the household index cases with ETEC (ST and ST/LT) diarrhoea. The use of such water in food preparation as well as for drinking was implicated by the authors. *E. coli* were found to be a common and important contaminant of local weaning foods, which, as in The Gambia, were worse in this respect than more adult type foods such as boiled rice. The proportion of a weanling child's food samples containing *E. coli* was significantly related to the number of attacks of ETEC diarrhoea experienced in one year (Black et al 1982b). No similar correlation could be demonstrated with respect to *E. coli*-containing drinking water supplies. This was probably due, at least in part, to a dose effect — the number of organisms being ingested from a food source far outweighing the contribution from a drinking water source. Further confirmation of this point comes from a study by Watkinson et al (1981) indicating that even though organisms multiplied in glucose-electrolyte solutions prepared for oral rehydration therapy, daily consumption from such a source was likely to be insignificant compared with that derived from food.

Though it has been proposed that food is a more important source of bacterial contamination than drinking water in The Gambia, it would be unwise to extrapolate this uncritically to other parts of the globe. In an investigation into the microbiological qualities of the surface waters serving the city of Jakarta (Fig. 4.4), Gracey and co-workers (1979) found these to be so polluted as to resemble raw colonic contents with very high isolation rates of *Salmonellae* and other pathogens. This degree of faecal contamination of water is of a quite different order to that described in The Gambia (Barrell & Rowland 1979a) and is presumably related to the population concentration of a dirty, overcrowded, tropical city and the even greater opportunities for polluting surface waters as compared with wells. In the far less unhygienic environment of Perth, Western Australia, a recent study showed 10 per cent of acute gastroenteritis cases in young children to be associated with enterotoxigenic *Aeromonas* spp., a pathogen conventionally regarded as water-borne (Gracey et al 1982, Burke et al 1983).

Until now this section has been largely confined to reference to those bacterial organisms conventionally considered in the context of acute gastroenteritis. However, studies in The Gambia (Barrell & Rowland 1979b) documented the presence of other potential food-poisoning organisms such

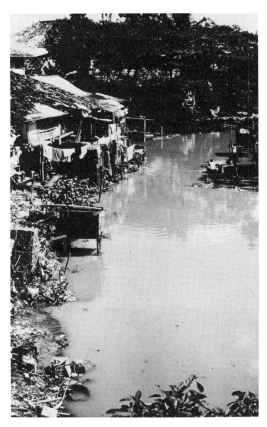

Fig. 4.4 Polluted surface waters in overcrowded urban slums. (From Gracey et al 1979, with permission of The Editor of Transactions of the Royal Society of Tropical Medicine and Hygiene)

as *B. cereus*, *Staphylococcus aureus* and *Clostridium welchii*. Surprisingly, the contribution of such organisms and pathology to endemic childhood diarrhoea in the third world is not known. However, there is no reason to believe that this is insignificant and may account for some. of the many episodes of diarrhoea in which no conventional pathogen is isolated from the stools.

In addition to gastroenteritis and food-poisoning a third aetiological concept should be considered at this point. Reference has been made earlier to the weanling diarrhoea sydrome. This denotes a pattern of recurring or relapsing diarrhoea commonly seen in individual children where diarrhoeal prevalence in the community is high. In the original description by Gordon et al in 1963 the association with malnutrition was noted, as was the frequent failure to identify pathogenic organisms, admittedly without the benefit of recent advances in knowledge of aetiology and techniques for identification of 'newer' pathogens.

The precise nature of the weaning diarrhoea syndrome is still ill-understood but microbial contamination of the proximal bowel almost certainly plays a role. This is a phenomenon now widely described in severely malnourished children whereby the bacterial flora of the oropharynx (Gracey et al 1973a) and the gut (Mata et al 1972, Gracey et al 1973b, Heyworth & Brown 1975) tends to reflect that of the contaminated environment in which such children commonly exist. This phenomenon is not restricted to malnourished children nor are the pathological consequences entirely clear (Rowland et al 1981) but in those instances where toxin-producing enteric organisms have been identified in jejunal fluid there is no reason to doubt their pathogenicity. Further insight into this problem comes from Swedish workers who found in food, both in their own country and in Ethiopia, considerable numbers of enteric organisms not conventionally listed as diarrhoeal pathogens, such as *Pseudomonas, Klebsiella, Proteus* and *Enterobacter* which they subsequently demonstrated to be capable of producing enterotoxins (Jiwa et al 1981). These bacteria are included in the long list of those documented in the studies above where systematic identification has been carried out on small bowel contaminants. The pathophysiological aspects of this syndrome have been discussed in Chapter 2.

No single study of endemic diarrhoea in children in underpriviledged communities has ever covered all these aetiological possibilities at the same time, perhaps because of logistic and financial constraints, so that the implications of these disparate findings are largely speculative; nor are priorities readily assigned. If these various mechanisms are all of real public health importance, then the major role of food hygiene and also of water is readily appreciated in the context of diarrhoeal illness with its attendant consequences on growth in early childhood.

SUMMARY

Diarrhoeal diseases are probably the major cause of non-dietary growth faltering in young children in developing countries. Some eminent workers have suggested that control of endemic diarrhoea would radically reduce the amount of early childhood malnutrition to the extent that specific nutritional measures would rarely be required. Our knowledge of the aetiology, and hence the epidemiology, of these diarrhocas is incomplcte but it is likely that bacterial pathogens are of overriding importance whether as agents of gastroenteritis, of food poisoning or of small bowel contamination. In the polluted domestic environment of many third world children there is abundant evidence for the opportunity of acquiring these gastrointestinal infections, food and water providing two of the most obvious and ubiquitous routes. The challenge of how to control this situation remains to be faced and aspects of this will be discussed in subsequent chapters.

REFERENCES

Barrell R A E, Rowland M G M 1979a The relationship between rainfall and well-water pollution in a West African (Gambian) village. Journal of Hygiene, Cambridge 83: 143–150

Barrell R A E, Rowland M G M 1979b Infant foods as a potential source of diarrhoeal illness in rural West Africa. Transactions of the Royal Society of Medicine and Hygiene 73: 85–90

Barrell R A E, Rowland M G M 1980 Commercial milk products and indigenous weaning foods in a rural West African environment: a bacteriological perspective. Journal of Hygiene, Cambridge 84: 191–202

Black R E, Brown K H, Becker S 1983 Influence of acute diarrhea on the growth parameters of children. In: Bellanti J A (ed) Acute diarrhea: its nutritional consequences in children. Nestlé Nutrition Workshop Series, Vol 2. Raven Press, New York, p 75–84

Black R E, Brown K H, Becker S, Alim A R M A, Huq I 1982a Longitudinal studies of infectious diseases and physical growth of children in rural Bangladesh 11. Incidence of diarrhea and association with known pathogens. American Journal of Epidemiology 115: 315–324

Black R E, Brown K H, Becker S, Alim A R M A, Merson M H 1982b Contamination of weaning foods and transmission of enterotoxigenic Escherichia coli diarrhoea in children in rural Bangladesh. Transactions of the Royal Society of Tropical Medicine and Hygiene, 76: 259–264

Black R E, Brown K H, Becker S, Yunus M 1982c Longitudinal studies of infectious diseases and physical growth of children in rural Bangladesh 1. Patterns of morbidity. American Journal of Epidemiology 115: 305–314

Black R E, Merson M H, Rowe B, Taylor P R, Alim A R M A, Gross R J, Sack D A 1981 Enterotoxigenic Escherichia coli diarrhoea: acquired immunity and transmission in an endemic area. Bulletin of the World Health Organization 59: 263–268

Burke V, Gracey M, Robinson J, Peck D, Beaman J, Bundell C The microbiology of childhood gastroenteritis: Aeromonas species and other infective agents. Journal of Infectious Diseases 148: 68–74

Chung A W 1948 The effect of oral feeding at different levels on the absorption of foodstuffs in infantile diarrhea. Journal of Pediatrics 33: 1–13

Gordon J E, Chitkara I D, Wyon J B 1963 Weanling diarrhea. American Journal of Medical Science 245: 345–377

Gracey M, Burke V, Robinson J 1982 Aeromonas-associated gastroenteritis. Lancet ii: 1304–1306

Gracey M, Ostergaard P, Adnan S W, Iveson J B 1979 Faecal pollution of surface waters in Jakarta. Transactions of the Royal Society of Tropical Medicine and Hygiene 73 (3): 306–308

Gracey M, Stone D E, Suharjono, Sunoto 1973a Oropharyngeal microflora in malnourished children. Australian Paediatric Journal 9: 260–262

Gracey M, Suharjono, Sunoto, Stone D E 1973b Microbial contamination of the gut: another feature of malnutrition. American Journal of Clinical Nutrition 26: 1170–1174

Heyworth B, Brown J 1975 Jejunal microflora in malnourished Gambian children. Archives of Disease in Childhood 50: 27–33

Hoyle B, Yunus M, Chen L C 1980 Breast-feeding and food intake among children with acute diarrheal disease. American Journal of Clinical Nutrition 33: 2365–2371

Jiwa S F, Krovacek K, Wadström T 1981 Enterotoxigenic bacteria in food and water from an Ethiopian community. Applied Environmental Microbiology 41: 1010–1019

Martinez C, Chavez A 1979 The effect of nutritional status on the frequency and severity of infections. Nutrition Reports International 19 (3): 307–314

Mata L J 1978 The children of Santa Maria Cauqué: A prospective field study of health and growth. The MIT Press, Cambridge, Massachusetts & London, England, p 395

Mata L J, Jiminez F, Cordon M, Rosales R, Prera E, Schneider R E, Viteri E 1972 Gastrointestinal flora of children with protein calorie malnutrition. American Journal of Clinical Nutrition 25: 1118–1126

Mata L J, Kronmal R A, Garcìa B, Butler W, Urrutia J J, Murillo S 1976 Breast-feeding, weaning and the diarrhoeal syndrome in a Guatemalan Indian village. In: Elliott K (ed) Acute diarrhoea in childhood. Ciba Foundation Symposium 42 (New Series). Amsterdam Elsevier/Excerpta Medica/North-Holland, Amsterdam, p 311–338

Mata L J, Kronmal R A, Urrutia J J, Garcìa B 1977 Effect of infection on food intake and the nutritional state: perspectives as viewed from the village. American Journal of Clinical Nutrition 30: 1215–1227

Molla A M, Molla Ayesha, Sarker S A, Rahaman M M 1983 Food intake during and after recovery from diarrhea in children. In: Chen L C, Scrimshaw N S (eds) Diarrhea and malnutrition. Interactions, mechanisms, and interventions. Plenum Press, New York & London, p 113–123

Molla Ayesha, Molla A M, Khatun M 1984 Effect of nutritional status of children on intake and absorption of nutrients. In: Eekels R, Ransome-Kuti O (eds) Child health in the tropics. Sixth Nutricia Symposium. Martinus-Nijhof Publishers, The Hague, in press

Palmer D L, Koster F T, Alam A K M J, Islam M R 1976 Nutritional status: a determinanat of the severity of diarrhea in patients with cholera. Journal of Infectious Diseases 134 (1): 8–14

Park E A 1924 Newer viewpoints in infant feeding. Proceedings of Connecticut State Medical Society p 190

Rosenberg I H 1978 Resumé of the discussion on 'Direct nutritional interventions'. American Journal of Clinical Nutrition 11: 2083–2088.

Rowland M G M 1982 Epidemiology of childhood diarrhea in The Gambia. In: Chen L C, Scrimshaw N S (eds) Diarrhea and malnutrition. Interactions, mechanisms, and interventions. Plenum Press, New York & London, p 87–98

Rowland M G M, Cole T J, Whitehead R G 1977 A quantitative study into the role of infection in determining nutritional status in Gambian village children. British Journal of Nutrition 37: 441–450

Rowland M G M, Cole T J, McCollum J P K 1981 Weanling diarrhoea in The Gambia: implications of a jejunal intubation study. Transactions of the Royal Society of Tropical Medicine and Hygiene 75 (2): 215–218

Rowland M G M, Whitehead R G 1980 The epidemiology of protein-energy malnutrition in children in a West African village community: A summary of the work of the M R C Dunn Nutrition Group 1974–1978. Medical Research Council, London. p 70

Sack R B 1983 Bacterial and parasitic agents of acute diarrhea. In: Bellanti J A (ed) Acute diarrhea: its nutritional consequences in children. Nestlé Nutrition Workshop Series, vol 2. Raven Press, New York, p 53–65

Scrimshaw N S, Taylor C E, Gordon J E 1968 Interactions of nutrition and infection. World Health Monograph Series No 57, Geneva, p 329

Snyder J D, Merson M H 1982 The magnitude of the global problem of acute diarrhoeal disease: a review of active surveillance data. Bulletin of the World Health Organization 60 (4): 605–613

Watkinson M, Lloyd-Evans N, Watkinson A M 1981 The use of oral glucose-electrolyte solution prepared with untreated well water in acute non-specific childhood diarrhoea. Transactions of the Royal Society of Tropical Medicine and Hygiene 74: 657–662

Wray J D 1978 Direct nutrition intervention and the control of diarrheal disease in pre-school children. American Journal of Clinical Nutrition 11: 2073–2082

Viral diarrhoeas

INTRODUCTION

Acute diarrhoeal disease has long been recognized as an important public health problem throughout the world and is the major cause of hospital attendance and admission in developing countries. The highest percentage of diarrhoeal illness is in children below 2 years of age and it has been estimated that in developing countries it is responsible for 30 per cent of deaths in infants. The distribution of diarrhoeal diseases varies from one country to another and national data on morbidity and mortality from several South-East Asian countries were presented recently in Australia (Mackenzie 1982).

Recent evidence has indicated that viruses are responsible for the majority of diarrhoeal episodes in infants and young children in both developed and developing countries and may cause a considerable extent of malnutrition due to associated malabsorption. During the past decade, the diagnostic use of electron microscopy (EM) directly on specimens of faeces has shown viruses to be present in the acute stage of disease, and it is now possible to assign a viral aetiology to many diarrhoeal episodes in infants, young children and even adults. Rotaviruses have been the most commonly observed virus, but several other candidate aetiological agents are also known or suspected (Lam 1982). These include Norwalk and related viruses, adenoviruses, astroviruses, caliciviruses, coronaviruses and small round structured and non-structured viruses. Evidence is accumulating that some of these agents can cause diarrhoea, but the role of the others is still uncertain.

Viruses involved in diarrhoea

We have divided the now considerable list of viruses associated with diarrhoea into two sections: those mostly associated with endemic diarrhoea and those associated with epidemics (Table 5.1). As will become apparent, this distinction is far from being absolute but the division may have practical value for those concerned with investigating the condition. Those viruses listed under endemic diarrhoea are more likely to be found in sporadic cases where there is little to suggest a common source while those listed under

Table 5.1 Viruses associated with gastroenteropathy

	No. of serotypes at present
Endemic diarrhoea	
Rotavirus	4
Astrovirus	4
Adenovirus, fastidious	3
Coronavirus	1
Calicivirus (some)	1
Epidemic diarrhoea	
Norwalk	3
Calicivirus (some)	2
Small round viruses (SRVs)	unknown
Small round structured viruses (SRSVs)	unknown
Adenovirus, fastidious	unknown

epidemic diarrhoea are less likely to be identified in individual stools. This may be due more to their lack of clear identifying features to make their recognition certain and evidence from several cases may be necessary before their involvement can be recognized.

The main exception to this division is the caliciviruses. These have been included under both headings as they may be found both sporadically and in outbreaks. Their association with disease, however, has been found to be more clear-cut in outbreaks of diarrhoea and vomiting.

Although it is possible to identify the morphological type of most of these viruses with some certainty, they are not all equally easy to recognize. From the evidence gathered over the last 10 years, we now know that rotaviruses can be recognized with ease in the electron microscope and this is due to their size, characteristic appearance, and the frequency of infections with them. The relative importance of the various viruses is still being established and investigators should keep an open mind meantime.

ENDEMIC DIARRHOEA

Rotaviruses

Human rotavirus infection was first detected in Melbourne, Australia, in 1973 by thin-section electron microscopic examination of duodenal biopsies obtained from children with acute diarrhoea. Shortly after this discovery, the virus was seen by electron microscopy of diarrhoeal stool specimens in Australia, Canada, the United Kingdom and the USA (Fig. 5.1a). The complete virus is 70 nm in size, contains a segmented genome of 11 pieces of double-stranded RNA, and has an inner and outer capsid. The International Committee for Taxonomy of Viruses has classified it as a genus within the family Reoviridae.

Rotaviruses have emerged as the commonest virus to be associated with diarrhoea in infants and young children ill enough to require admission to hospital. Because of the important role rotaviruses play in diarrhoeal ill-

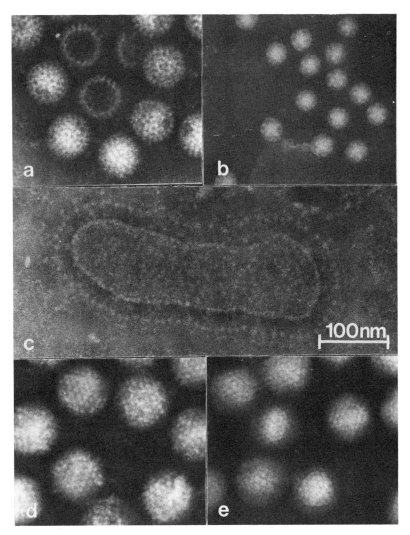

Fig. 5.1 The viruses associated mostly with endemic diarrhoea. **a**. Rotavirus. **b**. Astrovirus.
c. Coronavirus. **d**. Adenovirus from stool by direct electron microscopy. **e**. Adenovirus type
2 from cell culture, for comparison. All viruses printed at a final magnification of 200 000
×. Scale bar 100 nm. Negative contrast with 3% potassium phosphotungstate, pH 7.0.

nesses, this subject was reviewed in depth by a WHO Scientific Working
Group in 1980 (WHO 1980) and again in 1982 (WHO 1983).

Rotavirus infection probably spreads by faecal-oral transmission, a view
supported by volunteer and animal experiments. The relative importance
of other mechanisms of spread (water, food, air and fomites) has yet to be
elucidated and factors such as climate, humidity, overcrowding and cultural
habits also influence the incidence of rotavirus infection.

Surveys of the prevalence of antibodies to rotavirus in tropical as well as temperate countries have shown them to be very common in newborn babies due to transfer of maternal antibody. This prevalence falls in the first 6 months of life but becomes very high again by the age of 2–3 years. There is evidence that antibodies are acquired at an earlier age in children from developing countries. This rapid acquisition of rotavirus antibodies parallels that observed with respiratory syncytial and parainfluenza 3 viruses. In temperate countries rotavirus infections have been found to be more common in the colder season whereas there is less correlation with seasonal variations in tropical areas.

Nosocomial infections due to rotaviruses are not uncommon in developed countries and several reports have been published on outbreaks in many hospital nurseries for the newborn. Epidemics of rotavirus infection have also been observed in closed communities such as nursing homes, day care centres and kindergartens. Children in developing countries are particularly susceptible to mixed infections, e.g. rotavirus with *E. coli*, *Salmonella*, *Shigella*, *Campylobacter*, protozoa and other enteric viruses and this may contribute to the severity of cases in these regions. Animal experiments have shown that mixed infection with rotavirus and *E. coli* is likely to result in a more severe infection than either pathogen alone.

Serotypes

Sequential infections with human rotavirus have been documented in infants and young children, suggesting that there is more than one serotype. Immune electron microscopy and serum neutralization tests showed considerable diversity among rotaviruses. Differences between human strains were detected using complement-fixation (CF), enzyme-linked immunosorbent assay (ELISA), immune adherence haemagglutination (IAHA) and by serum neutralization using a fluorescent focus reduction method. There was considerable confusion in the literature because each worker used a different numbering system for the various serotypes.

There is now general agreement that rotaviruses distinguished on the basis of their neutralization by hyperimmune sera should be referred to as serotypes. Such serotypes are defined by differences in the polypeptides specified by the ninth genomic segment of the viral ribonucleic acid (RNA). Rotaviruses distinguished serologically by CF, ELISA or IAHA should be described as subgroups and are based on differences in the major inner capsid polypeptide which is specified by the sixth genomic segment. Based on the above criteria, two subgroups of rotaviruses have been reported and at least four serotypes of the virus infecting man can be differentiated.

The World Health Organization (WHO) has recommended the adoption of the serotyping nomenclature as designated by the WHO Collaborating Centre for Human Rotaviruses in Birmingham, United Kingdom (1984), and to avoid further confusion, it further recommends that all potential new types be sent to this Centre to be evaluated and assigned a serotype number.

The difficulty of cultivating human rotaviruses in tissue culture has impeded the definition of serotypes among these viruses. This difficulty has, fortunately, been largely overcome. Direct isolation of human rotaviruses from stool specimens from patients with diarrhoea has been reported using roller cultures of MA-104 (Sato et al 1981, Urasawa et al 1981) and in primary cynomolgus monkey kidney cells (Hasegawa et al 1982) in the presence of trypsin. It should now become easier to establish serotypes using conventional assays. A more rapid method for determining both the subgroup and serotype of rotaviruses in faeces from patients has been described, using an ELISA reaction with suitably absorbed sera (Thouless et al 1982).

Differences in the electrophoretic mobility of the 11 genomic segments of the virus RNA have also been used to differentiate rotaviruses and could serve as an important tool for epidemiological studies. Human rotaviruses can be broadly separated into two groups (electrophoretypes) with the 'short' pattern in subgroup 1 and the 'long' pattern in subgroup 2 (Kalica et al 1981) (Fig. 5.2).

Recently, morphologically typical rotaviruses have been found in Australia (Rodger et al 1982) and France (Nicolas et al 1983) which do not cross-react serologically with other strains. In particular they lack the group antigen and similar strains have also been recovered from pigs, calves and chickens. So far, these strains appear to be rare but they cause diagnostic problems as they will not be detected by present antibody-based tests, only by EM. They have been referred to as pararotaviruses but this may be misleading because there is as yet no evidence that they differ from other rotaviruses in any important way.

Studies have suggested that rotavirus can be associated with respiratory diseases in infants and young children. A recent report by Yolken & Murphy (1982) has indicated that some cases of sudden infant death syndrome are also associated with rotavirus infection but further research will be needed to establish the significance of this.

Astroviruses

Where a comparison has been made (in Glasgow), astroviruses are associated with diarrhoea in childhood by evidence which parallels closely that for rotaviruses (Madeley 1983). Approximately 80 per cent of astroviruses were seen in the stools of children with diarrhoea in which the astrovirus was the only potential pathogen observed. In another 10 per cent, the astrovirus was associated with another virus, was not the first virus observed or was observed too late after onset for the association to be convincing. In the remaining 10 per cent, the child's gut function appeared to be perfectly

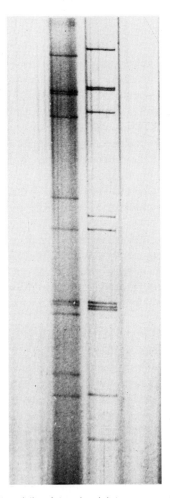

Fig. 5.2 'Short' (on the left) and 'long' (on the right) patterns of rotavirus RNA segments
in polyacrylamide gel electrophoresis. The specimens were stool extracts run in parallel and
the gel was stained by a silver impregnation method. Note that both strains of the virus
show 11 segments (in the long pattern segments 2 and 3 have run very close to each other)
but the distance migrated by each segment is not always the same with the two strains.
Basically, subgroup 1 strains show 'short' patterns and subgroup 2 strains show 'long'
patterns, but there are numerous other differences between strains that are still under study.
(Gel prepared and photographed by Dr R B Moosai, University of Newcastle upon Tyne.)

normal. Very similar proportions were observed with rotaviruses in the same
area and the main difference between the two viruses was the frequency with
which they were observed. Rotaviruses were found between three and four
times as frequently but the evidence of pathogenic potential was similar for
both viruses. Nonetheless, astroviruses have been reported by comparatively
few laboratories and their distribution and importance worldwide has yet
to be determined.

Morphologically similar viruses have now been observed in the faeces of lambs and calves in whom natural infection was often, but not invariably, associated with diarrhoea.

Astroviruses are small spherical viruses about 28 nm in diameter. When present in faeces they may be found in very large numbers indeed and not infrequently in a crystalline array (Fig. 5.1b). They have been so called because a proportion have a five- or six-pointed star on the surface. The particles have a smooth circular outline and stain-penetrated ('empty') particles are uncommon. They were originally described in 1975 and were of a morphological type that had not been observed before. It is probable that they contain RNA.

There is now published evidence for at least two serotypes of human astroviruses and it is probable that there are at least four (Lee & Kurtz, personal communication). As far as is known at present, astroviruses do not possess a group antigen and each serotype is distinct. The separate serotypes have been identified by the use of immunofluorescence in which each serotype does not react with antiserum to any of the other serotypes.

Astroviruses do not grow in routine cell cultures, but at least two serotypes (Spinage and Magowan) have been adapted to serial passage in human embryo kidney (HEK) and LLC-MK2 cells by the use of trypsin (Lee & Kurtz 1981).

Volunteer experiments in adults have shown that it is possible to infect them with astrovirus but the effects are mild. Nevertheless, virus is excreted in considerable quantities and most of the volunteers seroconverted (Kurtz et al 1979). In this, they parallel rotaviruses closely with which similar experiments in adults have also yielded little evidence of illness. We do not yet know whether the different serotypes vary in their virulence.

One serological survey has been published (Kurtz & Lee 1978). Although the numbers were small, the pattern of acquisition of antibody was similar to that with rotaviruses with 71 per cent having antibody by the age of 4 years.

Coronaviruses

Coronaviruses are worldwide in distribution and are known to cause a variety of serious infections in animals, including gastroenteritis. Their role as human pathogens is less certain although several strains have been isolated in association with upper respiratory tract infection of man. Thus far, attempts to associate them with gastroenteritis have yielded conflicting results.

Workers in Vellore in Southern India first reported particles with fringes resembling coronaviruses in human faeces in 1974. These particles are 40–800 nm in size, markedly pleomorphic and have a fringe (approximately 18–22 nm in length) surrounding them (Fig. 5.1c). There are some morphological differences between the coronovirus particles seen in faecal samples and those of human respiratory coronaviruses. Antigenic cross-reactivity between these two groups has not been demonstrated and they are often difficult to distinguish clearly from cellular and other debris in stools.

Human enteric coronaviruses have now been seen in stool samples obtained from Australian Aborigines and patients with acute diarrhoea in the UK. However, their pathogenicity has not yet been determined. In Southern India, these particles have a wide prevalence in faecal samples obtained from chronic diarrhoea and malabsorption and they are often excreted for months. The slow progress in characterizing coronaviruses and establishing an association with diarrhoeal diseases is largely due to the difficulties in growing them in cell or organ cultures. The majority of coronaviruses have shown no evidence of growth in cell culture, the possible exceptions being the reported growth of a UK strain in organ cultures (Caul & Clarke 1975, Caul & Egglestone 1977). Recently, however, coronavirus has been seen in faeces of neonates from an outbreak of necrotizing enterocolitis in France (Sureau et al 1980) but it is possible that this is a calf strain (Patel et al 1982).

The role of coronavirus in both acute and chronic intestinal disease in man is still very undefined. It is important to confirm the isolation of these viruses in cell culture and to determine whether these viruses are truly of human origin or merely cross-infection of man by animal coronaviruses.

Identification of coronaviruses is particularly difficult by EM and a more objective and reliable method is needed. An ELISA system has been used in the diagnosis of acute respiratory infection in children caused by human coronaviruses (Macnaughton et al 1983) and might be adapted to the detection of these viruses in diarrhoeal stools.

Adenoviruses

Adenoviruses are observed in approximately 5 per cent of routine childhood stools in the temperate zones where surveys have been made. Only a proportion of these have been observed in diarrhoeal stools and it is not yet clear whether the adenovirus caused the disease observed. Since few of such recognizates can be typed, it is not even possible to say whether some serotypes have greater virulence than others.

Several outbreaks have been associated with adenoviruses but here the evidence is confusing. The earliest to be reported was in a long-stay children's ward (Flewett et al 1975) in which a number of children had diarrhoea and adenovirus was observed in the stools of a proportion. The virus resisted all attempts in a number of laboratories to grow it in cell culture but evidence obtained by immune electron microscopy suggested that it might be a type 7. In two other outbreaks adenoviruses were the only potential pathogens to be recognized (Whitelaw et al 1977, Richmond et al 1979). Again no virus was isolated in cell culture.

A considerable number of adenovirus serotypes have been recovered from faeces in cell cultures, including most of those associated with respiratory disease. There has been little convincing evidence to link these isolates with episodes of diarrhoea and the very occasional outbreak involving adenovirus type 7, for example, did not suggest that it was a significant gut pathogen. With the advent of electron microscopic examination of stool extracts, it became apparent that a considerable number of infections were not being identified by cell culture. Soon, a paradox emerged that the chances of isolating an adenovirus from stool was in inverse proportion to the amount of virus detected by electron microscopy (EM). These hitherto unrecognized adenoviruses were typical morphologically and there has been no reason to doubt that they are true adenoviruses (Fig. 5.1d and e). There is now evidence (de Jong et al 1981, 1983) that these fastidious adenoviruses form at least two new serotypes. These have been provisionally allocated numbers 40 and 41 and it is possible there is a subtype (41a) of type 41 (Kidd et al 1983). The original proposal to call fastidious adenoviruses type 38 (de Jong et al 1981) has been superseded by these new proposals and it is likely that the designation 38 will be applied to a new respiratory adenovirus. With active research still continuing, it is likely that additional serotypes will be added later. Two that have been identified appear to possess the group antigen common to all human mastadenoviruses. Treatment of extracted DNA with restriction endonucleases has yielded fragments which are different from those found in the previously known serotypes.

The term 'fastidious' has been used to describe these new adenoviruses rather than 'non-growing' because some grow, although not well, in cell types not used routinely in diagnostic laboratories. Their failure to grow is therefore not necessarily absolute but no one has yet discovered the key to growing them routinely. The alternative of 'enteric' is also misleading as the previously recognized types may also be recovered from the gut.

With several of the EM detectable stool viruses, animal diarrhoeal disease associated with morphologically indistinguishable viruses is known. This is not so with adenoviruses, where no animal parallels have been described. No volunteer experiments have been reported either and this may be due to the difficulties of identifying particular serotypes — without clear identification it would be impossible to do satisfactory experiments. Further progress will have to await a reliable identification system.

EPIDEMIC DIARRHOEA

Norwalk and related viruses

Norwalk was originally identified by IEM in an outbreak of diarrhoea and vomiting in a primary school in Norwalk, Ohio (Blacklow et al 1972). It has also been recognized in a number of other common source outbreaks, mostly in America. Serological surveys, however, have shown that the virus is not exclusive to the USA. One such survey in the USA (Greenberg & Kapikian 1978) has shown that antibody is gradually acquired with age and that by the age of 50 most of those investigated had detectable levels of antibody. The rate of acquisition was much slower than for rotavirus or astrovirus and suggests that the virus is much less prevalent among children and young adults, at least in the US. This would be consistent with it causing occasional outbreaks with the victims being of any age and not predominantly children.

A similar survey in Bangladesh (Black et al 1982) has confirmed the presence of the virus but antibody is acquired much earlier. By the age of 5 years, more than half the children studied had developed antibody but here too, acquisition of Norwalk antibody lagged behind that of rotavirus, although the interval was shorter.

Norwalk and its related viruses (Montgomery County and Hawaii) appear to affect adults as well as children. In the original Norwalk outbreak, adults as well as the children in the school were affected and two related viruses were recovered from family outbreaks affecting both adults and children.

Norwalk virus has proved a difficult virus to visualize in the EM and for some time the micrographs of the virus, all obtained after addition of acute or convalescent serum obtained from patients, were thought to represent a small 27 nm particle with antibody. It now seems likely that the virus itself has an irregular, almost 'hairy' surface structure, somewhat similar to that produced by antibody. However, on some particles (Fig. 5.3a) there is a suggestion of a definite surface structure where the elements are too large to be due to antibody. It now seems likely that Figure 5.3a represents virus with no antibody coating it, and that the original description of this virus as a parvovirus is incorrect. In addition, it is also likely that the previously quoted size is too low and the true size lies in the range of 30–35 nm. There is now evidence that the virions contain RNA and that the virus structure is almost entirely assembled from a single polypeptide. These are both features similar to those of caliciviruses (Studdert 1978) but the published value for the size of the polypeptide is lower than that for known caliciviruses and the possibility that Norwalk is really a calicivirus has still to be confirmed.

Norwalk and Montgomery County are antigenically related but Hawaii appears to be distinct. Morphologically similar viruses have been observed in other countries, including the UK and Australia, and associated with outbreaks of diarrhoea and vomiting. Where they have been investigated, they do not cross-react with Norwalk, but may prove to be part of the same genus when more is known about them. Their lack of clearly identifying features makes it difficult to be certain about this at present.

The most unexpected finding about Norwalk has come from experiments using adult volunteers (Parrino et al 1977). Twelve of them were infected using a bacteria-free filtrate of a stool extract. Six became ill and developed antibody in serum and in aspirated duodenal juice. Some two to three years later, the same 12 subjects were challenged again and the 6 who were ill the

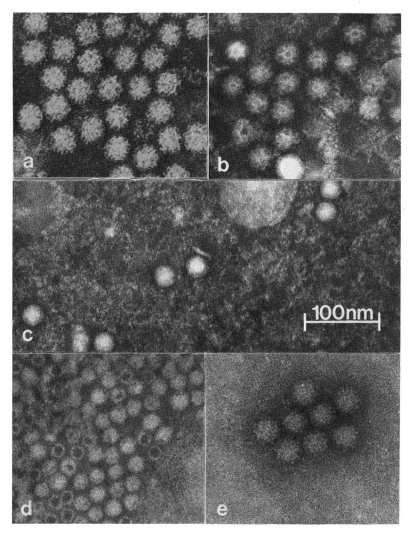

Fig. 5.3 The viruses associated mostly with epidemic diarrhoea and/or vomiting.
a. Norwalk virus. **b.** Calicivirus. **c.** Small round viruses (SRVs). **d.** Parvovirus: note empty particles and the hexagonal outline of some of the virions. **e.** Small round structured viruses (SRSVs): compare with SRVs and note the surface 'hairiness' of these. This is not due to antibody. All viruses printed at a final magnification of 200 000 ×. Scale bar 100 nm. Negative contrast with 3% potassium phosphotungstate pH 7.0. (Micrograph of Norwalk reproduced from Kapikian et al 1972 Journal of Virology 10: 1075, by kind permission of the authors and the Editor).

first time were ill again while the others remained well. Later, four of those who had been ill on two occasions were challenged a third time and one became ill yet again. The illnesses were mild but these results have clear implications for hopes of preventing infection by Norwalk or any of the other viruses by the use of vaccines.

Caliciviruses

Caliciviruses infecting cats, pigs and sealions and northern fur seals had been known for some time before human strains were recognized. They were first discovered in the faeces of children with sporadic diarrhoea and probably cause a small proportion of endemic cases. Perhaps, more importantly, they have now been linked with several outbreaks of 'winter-vomiting' in the UK and Japan (Cubitt et al 1979, Chiba et al 1979) and they have also been recorded in the USA and Canada. It is probable that they are distributed throughout the world. In the recorded outbreaks, most of the cases have been in children but some adults have also been affected. Outbreaks of vomiting have caused problems in diagnosis for years and a calicivirus should be considered a possible cause of any outbreak where vomiting is a particular feature.

In appearance, caliciviruses are 33–35 nm in diameter with a surface covered in regularly arranged hollows. These cause the periphery of the particle to appear ill-defined and may also give rise to a very characteristic six-pointed 'Star-of-David' arrangement (Fig. 5.3b). It may sound as if this six-pointed star may be confused with that of an astrovirus but a comparison of Figure 5.1b with Figure 5.3b will show that they are quite different. The points of similarity and difference between the two viruses have been discussed by Madeley (1979). Caliciviruses contain RNA and biochemical analysis of their structure shows that it is composed almost entirely of a single polypeptide. This has a molecular weight of about 60 000 and, since this is a feature not shared by other small RNA viruses, other viruses possessing a similar feature (e.g. Norwalk virus) may eventually also prove to be caliciviruses.

Three separate serotypes of human caliciviruses have been recognized by immune electron microscopy. Two of these (one in the UK and one in Japan) have been associated with outbreaks while the third, found in the UK, has been more associated with endemic diarrhoea. There appears to be little or no cross-reactivity between the strains, although it is difficult to be certain about this with the insensitive technique of IEM.

No volunteer studies with caliciviruses have yet been reported. A small serological survey carried out in Japan (Sakuma et al 1981) has shown a similar acquisition pattern of antibody with age to that found with rotaviruses and astroviruses. It would be useful to know if this antibody was protective.

Small round viruses (SRVs)

There are an appreciable number of other virus-like objects to be found in diarrhoeal stools and, less frequently, in normal stools as well. These may be divided into two morphological groups, small round viruses or SRVs and small round structured viruses or SRSVs, as indicated in Table 5.2. The main distinction between them is whether the virus particles show any sur-

Table 5.2 Small round viruses (SRVs) and small round structured viruses (SRSVs) found in stools

	Approximate size (nm)
SRVs	
Enteroviruses (polio, Coxsackie A & B, Echo)	25
Cockle[1]	22–25
Ditchling[2]	22–25
Parramatta[1]	22–25
Wollan[2]	22–25
Others[3]	22–25
Adeno-associated viruses	22
SRSVs	
Norwalk/Montgomery County	30–35
Hawaii	30–35
Taunton	30–35
Harlow	30–35
Others[4]	30–35

[1] Associated with food-borne outbreaks due to infected shellfish.
[2] Serologically related but not identical.
[3] Morphologically similar to other SRVs and observed in endemic diarrhoea. Their relation to the other SRVs, if any, is unknown.
[4] Do. for SRSVs, but may be associated with outbreaks.

face structure. The small round viruses (SRVs) appear to be featureless spheres with no surface structure and a clearly-defined entire edge. The others have an ill-defined edge and some surface structure (Caul & Appleton 1982).

SRVs

These do not have characteristic features, and this makes them difficult to identify. The certainty that they are viruses only grows with finding a considerable number of them, either in a single stool or in several stools from related cases. Where SRVs have been associated with outbreaks the number of stools examined has usually been small but their virus-like appearance and consistent size in the electron microscope has carried conviction. Because it is not always possible to investigate outbreaks thoroughly for viruses, it is likely that those involving SRVs are very much under-reported and in known episodes represent only a small fraction of the whole.

The SRVs can themselves be subdivided into two size classes although it is not yet clear whether these are indeed separate. The bigger ones are about 25 nm in diameter (Fig. 5.3c) and are indistinguishable from typical enteroviruses. Only rarely can an enterovirus be isolated from the same stool and it is possible that the others are atypical enteroviruses which fail to grow in routine cell culture. Enough diarrhoeal stool extracts have been inoculated into new born mice for it to be unlikely that they are Coxsackie A viruses which would not grow in cell cultures either. The smaller ones are about 20–22 nm in diameter and are similar in appearance to parvoviruses (Fig. 5.3d). Occasionally, they may be present in very large numbers and, under these circumstances, an adenovirus may also be found. These may be adeno-associated viruses and it is probable that these are different from other parvo-like viruses which are present in much smaller quantities and with no evidence of association with adenoviruses so far. The smaller SRVs have been associated with outbreaks of gastroenteropathy, some of which were most probably transmitted by shellfish as indicated in Table 5.2. They may also show an outline more hexagonal than round and it is not uncommon to find a considerable proportion of 'empty' particles. These features are seen in Figure 5.3d from a stool in which an adenovirus was also seen. These are therefore probably genuine parvoviruses.

As far as is known, most recognized SRVs are serologically distinct. The exceptions are Wollan and Ditchling (Table 5.2) which show some cross-reactivity by IEM (Appleton et al 1977). It is not, therefore, likely that any antibody-based tests (see under 3.2 below) will be available to investigate outbreaks.

No volunteer experiments or serological surveys have been reported nor has any evidence of growth in cell cultures been obtained. Consequently, there is no alternative at present to the electron microscope for investigating their association with disease.

SRSVs

SRSVs have mostly been recognized when they have been associated with outbreaks of gastroenteropathy. However, careful examination of stools from endemic diarrhoea has shown that similar viruses may be present in the community between epidemics (F J Bone, J Miller & C R Madeley, unpublished results). Where they have been involved in common-source outbreaks they may have been transmitted by food or water, although unequivocal evidence has yet to be obtained. In other cases no vehicle has been identified. No equivalent animal strains have yet been recognized although the possibility cannot be excluded.

The SRSVs differ from SRVs in having some evidence of surface structure. How this surface structure is arranged on the virus particle is not clearly visible by EM and it is not possible to say with certainty that they are a homogeneous group (Fig. 5.3e). They are about 35 nm in diameter but some variations in size have been reported. It is not yet clear whether these are true differences or whether they represent variations in measurement using different electron microscopes. It now seems unlikely that they are SRVs covered in antibody but the possibility that they may be the same as Norwalk and/or caliciviruses cannot yet be ruled out. Information about individual SRSVs is scanty at present.

Neither volunteer experiments nor serological surveys have been reported. No evidence for growth in cell cultures has been obtained either. The appearance of SRSVs has convinced several experienced electron microscopists that they are viruses and some, perhaps all, may yet prove to be caliciviruses. Although this may be so, in the absence of positive evidence it is necessary to keep an open mind and to record them separately.

DIAGNOSIS

Principles

The viruses listed above have no features in common. They vary in size, appearance, nucleic acid and antigenic structure. There is only one method of diagnosis that can be applied equally and simultaneously to all of them and that, as we shall see, has formidable limitations and drawbacks. This technique is electron microscopy and no other technique in diagnosis can match its versatility. In particular, it can be used to look for a 'new' virus when none of its attributes are known beforehand. However, the cost of it both in providing the machine and its skilled operation has meant that alternatives have been sought. With one exception — polyacrylamide gel electrophoresis of the RNA from rotavirus — all the alternative techniques depend on the use of specific antibody to find the virus. This has a number of important consequences which should be clearly understood.

The first is that a decision on which virus is to be sought has to be made before the test is started so that the appropriate antiserum (or kit) can be selected. The second is that where antisera are available, the test must be repeated on each stool extract for each virus. The third is that such antisera are available for only a small proportion of the possible viruses or their various serotypes of each one.

The practical consequences of these limitations is that antibody-based tests have been used more to investigate the role of individual viruses in gastroenteropathy rather than to investigate the condition as a whole. There is no doubt that such an approach may provide valuable information but may give a misleading impression of the relative importance of each of the viruses in this condition.

METHODS

Detection of virus or viral antigen

Electron microscopy

Virtually all virus recognizates have been made on stool extracts. Norwalk virus has been observed in vomit but only with difficulty, and other viruses have not been found. Although it is likely that at least some of the stool viruses can be transmitted through droplet-spread, no virus of any kind has been observed in respiratory secretions. Consequently, the specimen of choice for electron microscopy is a stool specimen.

Elaborate methods of separation of stool extract are not needed routinely and it is often possible to observe virus directly in an uncentrifuged or unconcentrated extract. Nevertheless, stool extracts contain large amounts of proteinaceous debris and salt which may be removed by differential high-speed centrifugation. Where a high-speed centrifuge is not available similar concentration may be achieved using polyacrylamide beads or pressure dialysis, although these latter two methods will remove less debris. The concentrated material can then be mixed with a negative stain (2–3% phosphotungstic acid at a neutral pH is probably the best all-round stain) and the mixture applied to a microscope grid. After drying it can be examined directly for virus particles. This is more difficult than it appears at first sight and all microscopists are not equally talented at finding virus.

The microscope must be a high resolution one and in good reliable order. Microscopes which are inconvenient to use, unstable or unreliable will yield very poor results. At best this technique is difficult to do well; technical difficulties will make it almost impossible.

It is essential that several examples of every virus observed are photographed, even when the operator is uncertain whether it is genuinely a virus. Such negatives can then be reviewed later and they provide the only objective evidence that a virus was found.

The sensitivity of the microscopy can be improved by the use of IEM. Antibody can be mixed with the stool extract to 'clump' the virus but this techniques should be used intelligently. Too much antibody will obscure the fine structure of the virus and may make it impossible to recognize. It may also aggregate the virus into such large clumps that they may fail to reach the grid at all. However, the technique may be used to help to identify the virus but, because naturally occurring clumps may be present anyway, such evidence should not be accepted too uncritically. It should also be remembered that the use of antibody to one virus will bias the results in favour of that virus and it is not uncommon to find more than one virus in a particular stool.

The second use of antibody is to coat the grids beforehand to provide a kind of adhesive for any of that virus in the extract. This, too, will bias the results in favour of the virus but may help to concentrate particles of that virus on the grid. This method, too, should be used only with a clear understanding of the implications of using it. The similar use of pooled human gamma-globulin gets round some of these objections but may increase the amount of other non-viral antigenic debris attracted to the grid.

The finding of one virus should not inhibit the operator from looking for a second one. It is quite common to find that more than one virus may be present and the second virus may differ very considerably in size and appearance from the first.

The principal advantage of electron microscopy is that it can detect a wide variety of viruses. In this it has no serious competitor. No prior decisions are necessary as to which virus is to be sought and any virus present in sufficient quantity can be recorded. However, electron microscopes are expensive to buy and to maintain. They are as liable to break down as any complicated piece of equipment and will require a skilled engineer to service and repair them. The operator must also be experienced, skilled, well-trained and talented! Each specimen must be examined individually for, on average, 15 minutes. It is insensitive, requiring not less than 10^6 particles/ml for even one to be detected. Nonetheless, where they are available and working they are an important tool in the investigation of diarrhoea.

Enzyme-linked immunosorbent assay

The ELISA system has been found to be a useful technique for the detection of rotaviruses and has been adopted by the WHO as the standard method for the detection of rotavirus antigen in stools. The WHO Collaborating Centre for human rotaviruses in Birmingham, UK, who developed the WHO ELISA kit for rotavirus, has field-tested the kit extensively and found it to be highly sensitive, specific and simple to perform. The kit has a reasonably long shelf life, is relatively stable under tropical conditions and, more important, it includes a confirmatory test for positive reactions. Whilst many groups have now developed ELISA systems for detecting rotavirus (including several which are commercially available), they do not all have reagents for confirming positive reactions, giving rise to false positive due very often to the presence of rheumatoid factor-like substances in faecal extracts.

The WHO ELISA kit is constantly being improved on to increase sensitivity, specificity, stability and reduce costs. A new kit is currently under development based on polyclonal and monoclonal antibodies respectively and involve the use of a cheaper enzyme and substrate for easier visual reading. There is a need to develop this technique for other enteric viruses.

Radioimmunoassay (RIA)

RIA and ELISA are two of the most sensitive techniques for the identification of gastroenteritis viruses. RIA systems for the detection of human rotavirus, Norwalk agent and enteric adenovirus in faeces have been reported. The test is relatively simple to perform and utilizes only small amounts of reagents. A large number of specimens can be tested in a single test. A variety of solid phases, including polystyrene beads, tissue culture tubes and microtitre plates have been used. An advantage of the microtitre system is that smaller volumes of valuable reagents are utilized but technical disadvantages include the use of expensive apparatus and the fact that the reagents have a short shelf-life and the radioactivity presents a biological hazard.

Other methods

Methods other than EM, ELISA and RIA for the detection of rotaviruses have been reviewed recently (Birch & Marshall 1983). These include counter-immunoelectrophoresis, complement-fixation, solid phase aggregation of coupled erthrocytes, reverse passive haemagglutination and latex agglutination. These tests have yet to establish themselves in the repertoire but the latex agglutination (Haikala et al 1983) and reverse passive haemagglutination (Nakagomi et al 1982) show some potential for widespread field application in developing countries, as being relatively cheap, stable and easy to use.

Detection of antibody

Serological diagnosis of viral diarrhoeas is not often performed because evidence is more easily obtained by direct examination of faeces. The main value of antibody tests has been in investigating the prevalence of various agents in particular populations and most of the methods mentioned above for rotavirus detection have also been adapted for antibody detection.

Research priorities

Although the past decade has seen much progress in our knowledge of viral diarrhoeas, there are still many priority areas for future research and these have been outlined in at least two publications (Report 1983, Holmes 1983). Data are available from numerous studies in both tropical and temperate countries on the monthly and annual frequency of rotavirus infection in children admitted to hospital, but there is still a need for long-term community-based studies of the incidence, prevalence and natural history of the infection, particularly in areas where rotavirus vaccine trials are planned. To this end the WHO Programme for Control of Diarrhoeal Diseases is funding several longitudinal studies of three years duration to determine mortality and morbidity rates for diarrhoea.

Further research is needed on the factors that influence the survival of rotaviruses and other viruses in the environment. The relative importance of water, food, air and fomites as vehicles in the spread of infection needs to be determined.

Further studies are also needed to demonstrate correlations between aspects of the immune response and protection, both for rotavirus and the other viral diarrhoeal agents. The importance of intestinal IgA rotavirus antibody needs to be confirmed and further investigated. More information is required on the kinetics and duration of local immune response (humoral and cellular) in persons of different ages and nutritional status.

The development of a rotavirus vaccine has been given a high priority and one of the major obstacles to this has been the difficulty in propagating human rotaviruses efficiently in cell cultures. This has largely been overcome and several human rotavirus strains have now been successfully cultivated in cynomolgus (long-tail macaca) monkey kidney or MA 104 cell cultures, or following reassortment with cultivable animal viruses. Yet another strategy being actively pursued is the utilization of a calf rotavirus as a human vaccine and a clinical trial is expected to take place shortly. Experimental animals should be sought in which human rotaviruses can induce diarrhoea beyond the early period of life. This would be important for studies of the safety and efficacy of candidate vaccines, and of the virulence of different strains.

It is encouraging to note that an international organization such as the WHO has created a special programme to study all aspects of diarrhoeal diseases (see Ch. 14). To date this programme is supporting some research projects in countries on all aspects of viral diarrhoea based on the priorities as listed above. It is envisaged that the next decade will see greater advances in our knowledge of viral diarrhoea, especially in the field of prevention and control.

REFERENCES

Appleton H, Buckley M, Thom B T, Cotton J L, Henderson S 1977 Virus-like particles in winter vomiting disease. Lancet i: 409–411
Birch C J, Marshall J A, 1983 Laboratory diagnosis of viral gastroenteritis. In: Lam S K (ed) Viral gastroenteritis. Asean Journal of Clinical Science Monograph II: 36–50
Black R E, Greenberg H B, Kapikian A Z, Brown K H, Becker S 1982 Acquisition of serum antibody in Norwalk virus and rotavirus and relation to diarrhoea in a longitudinal study of children in rural Bangladesh. Journal of Infectious Diseases 145: 483–489
Blacklow N R, Dolin R, Fedson, DuPont H L, Northrup R S, Horwick R B, Chanock R M 1972 Acute infectious non-bacterial gastroenteritis etiology and pathogenesis. Annals of Internal Medicine 76: 993–1008
Caul E O, Clarke S K R 1975 Coronaviruses propagated from a patient with non-bacterial gastroenteritis. Lancet ii: 853–854
Caul E O, Egglestone S I 1977 Further studies on human enteric coronaviruses. Archives of Virology 54: 107–117
Caul E O, Appleton H 1982 The electron microscopical and physical characteristics of small round human fecal viruses: an interim scheme for classification. Journal of Medical Virology 9: 257–265
Chiba S, Sakuma Y, Akihara M, Kogasaka R, Horino K, Nakao T, Fukui S 1979 An outbreak of gastroenteritis associated with calicivirus in an infant home. Journal of Medical Virology 4: 249–254
Cubitt W D, McSwiggan D A, Moore W 1979 Winter vomiting disease caused by calicivirus. Journal of Clinical Pathology 32: 786–793
de Jong J C, Wigand R, Kidd A H, Kapsenberg J G, Muzerie C J, Firtzlaff R, Wadell G 1981 Candidate adenovirus 38, associated with human infantile gastroenteritis and related to 'non-cultivable' enteric adenovirus. Abstracts of the Fifth International Congress of Virology, Strasbourg, P16/10
de Jong J C, Wigand R, Kidd A H, Wadell G, Kapsenberg J G, Muzerie C J, Wermenbol A G, Firtzlaff R G 1983 Candidate adenovirus 40 and 41: fastidious adenovirus from human infant stool. Journal of Medical Virology 11: 215–231
Flewett T H, Bryden A S, Davies H A, Morris C A 1975 Epidemic viral enteritis in a long stay children's ward. Lancet i: 4–5
Greenberg H B, Kapikian A Z 1978 Detection of Norwalk agent antibody and antigen by solid phase radioimmunoassay and immune adherence hemagglutination assay. Journal of the American Veterinary Medical Association 173: 620–623
Haikala O J, Kokkonen J O, Leinonen M K, Nurmi T, Mäntyjärvi R, Sarkkinen H K 1983 Rapid detection of rotavirus in stool by latex agglutination: comparison with

radioimmunoassay and electron microscopy and clinical evaluation of the test. Journal of Medical Virology 11: 91–97

Hasegawa A, Matsuno S, Inouye S ,Kono R, Tsurukubo Y, Mukoyama A, Saito Y 1982 Isolation of human rotaviruses in primary cultures of monkey kidney cells. Journal of Clinical Microbiology 16: 387–390

Holmes I H 1983 Viral gastroenteritis — research needs. In: Lam S K (ed) Viral gastroenteritis. Asean Journal of Clinical Science Monograph II: 51–53

Kalica A R, Greenberg H B, Espejo R T, Flores J, Wyatt R G, Kapikian A Z, Chanock R M 1981 Distinctive ribonucleic acid patterns of human rotavirus subgroups 1 and 2. Infection and Immunity 33: 958–961

Kidd A H, Banatvala J E, de Jong J C 1983 Antibodies to fastidious faecal adenoviruses (species 40 and 41) in sera from children. Journal of Medical Virology 11: 333–341

Kurtz J B, Lee T W 1978 Astrovirus gastroenteritis. Age distribution of antibody. Medical Microbiology and Immunology 166:227–230

Kurtz J B, Lee T W, Craig J W, Reed S E 1979 Astrovirus infection in volunteers. Journal of Medical Virology 3: 221–230

Lam S K 1982 Current concepts on aetiology and pathogenesis of diarrhoea caused by viruses. South-East Asian Journal of Tropical Medicine and Public Health 13: 325–330

Lee T W, Kurtz J B 1981 Serial propogation of astrovirus in tissue culture with the aid of trypsin. Journal of General Virology 57: 421–424

Mackenzie J S 1982 Viral diseases in South-East Asia and the Western Pacific. Academic Press, London, New York, San Francisco

Macnaughton M R, Flowers D, Isaacs D 1983 Diagnosis of human coronavirus infections in children using an enzyme-linked immunosorbent assay. Journal of Medical Virology 11: 319–325

Madeley C R 1979 A comparison of the features of astroviruses and caliciviruses seen in samples of faeces by electron microscopy. Journal of Infectious Diseases 139: 519–524

Madeley C R 1983 Viruses and diarrhoea: problems in proving causation. In: de la Maza L, Peterson E M (eds) Medical virology II. Elsevier Science Publishing Co Inc, New York, p 81–109

Nakagomi O, Nakagomi A, Suto T, Suzuki H, Kutsuzawa T, Tazawa F, Konno T, Ishida N 1982 Detection of human rotavirus by reversed passive hemagglutination (RPHA) using antibody against a cultivable human rotavirus as compared with electron microscopy (EM) and enzyme-linked immunosorbent assay (ELISA). Microbiology and Immunology 26: 747–751

Nicolas J C, Cohen J, Fortier B ,Lourenco M H, Bricout F 1983 Isolation of a human pararotavirus. Virology 124: 181–184

Parrino J A, Schreiber D S, Trier J S, Kapikian A Z, Blacklow N R 1977 Clinical immunity in acute gastroenteritis caused by Norwalk agent. New England Journal of Medicine 297: 86–89

Patel J R, Davies H A, Edington N, Laporte J, Macnaughton M R 1982 Infection of a calf with the enteric coronavirus strain, Paris. Archives of Virology 73: 319–327

Richmond S J, Caul E O, Dunn S M, Ashley C R, Clarke S K R, Seymour N R 1979 An outbreak of gastroenteritis in young children caused by adenovirus. Lancet i: 1178–1180

Rodger S M, Bishop R F, Holmes I H 1982 Detection of rotavirus-like agent associated with diarrhea in an infant. Journal of Clinical Microbiology 16: 724–726

Sakuma Y, Chiba S, Kogasaka R, Terashima H, Nakamura S, Horino K, Nakao T 1981 Prevalence of antibody to human calicivirus in general population of Northern Japan. Journal of Medical Virology 7: 221–225

Sato K, Inaba Y, Shinozaki T, Fugii R, Matsumoto M 1981 Isolation of human rotavirus in cell cultures. Archives of Virology 69: 155–160

Studdert M J 1978 Caliviruses — brief review. Archives of Virology 58: 157–191

Sureau C, Amiel-Tison C, Moscovici O, Lebon P, Laporte J, Chany C 1980 Une épidémie d'enterocolitis ulcéronécrosantes en maternité, arguments en faveur de son origine virale. Bulletin de l'Academie Nationale Médicale 164: 286–293

Thouless M, Beards G M, Flewett T H 1982 Serotyping and subgrouping of rotavirus strains by the ELISA test. Archives of Virology 73: 219–230

Urasawa T, Urasawa G, Taniguchi K 1981 Sequential passage of human rotavirus in MA-104 cells. Microbiology and Immunology 25: 1025–1035

Yolken R, Murphy M 1982 Sudden infant death syndrome associated with rotavirus infection. Journal of Medical Virology 10: 291–296

Whitelaw A, Davies H A, Parry J 1977 Electron microscopy of fatal adenovirus gastroenteritis. Lancet i: 361

World Health Organization 1980 Rotavirus and other viral diarrhoeas. Report of a WHO Scientific Working Group. Bulletin of the World Health Organization 58: 183–198

World Health Organization 1984 Nomenclature of human rotaviruses: designation of subgroups and serotypes. Bulletin of the World Health Organization 62: 501–503

Parasitic intestinal infections

INTRODUCTION

The parasitic diseases of the gastrointestinal tract associated with diarrhoea or malnutrition are related to poverty and ignorance. Infections with these organisms affect primarily undernourished populations that live in poor sanitary conditions and lack adequate education in hygiene. Most of these organisms are transmitted via soil contaminated with infected human faeces although several parasites may be acquired by ingestion of, or contact with, polluted water. Some of these protozoa and helminths are associated frequently with diarrhoea, others may cause diarrhoea under certain circumstances, while diarrhoea is not a feature of infection with a number of other organisms (Table 6.1).

In regions of the world where these parasites are common, multiple simultaneous infections of individuals are the rule rather than the exception. The effects of polyparasitism are often clinically inapparent, but in some

Table 6.1 Association of gastrointestinal parasitic infections with diarrhoea and their interactions with nutritional status

Organism	Association with diarrhoea	Nutrition impaired*	Disease influenced by malnutrition
Protozoa:			
Entamoeba histolytica	+ +	+	?
Giardia lamblia	+ +	+ +	?
Isospora belli	+	+ +	?
Balantidium coli	+	−	+
Helminths:			
Hookworms	±	+ +	?
Strongyloides stercoralis	+ +	+ +	+ +
Trichuris trichiura	±	−	?
Ascaris lumbricoides	−	?	?
Schistosoma sp.	±	±	−
Taenia sp	−	±	−

+ + common or severe + occasional or mild ± uncommon or minimal − nil ? uncertain
* Many patients have no impairment of nutrition; this table indicates severity that is reached in some individuals

situations they may either exacerbate clinical manifestations, or possibly suppress symptoms and signs of disease (Keusch & Migasena 1982). Consequently, it is difficult in many instances to dissect the relative roles of the various parasites in the genesis of both diarrhoea and malnutrition.

Two kinds of nutritional interactions may be seen in parasitic infections (Table 6.1). Firstly, they may impair nutritional status through a variety of mechanisms (Tomkins 1979, Rosenberg & Bowman 1982). Parasites may release substances which cause functional or structural changes in the intestinal mucosa, they may stimulate hypermotility, occasionally obstruct the pancreatic or bile ducts, and sometimes compete directly with the host for certain nutrients; the result is impaired digestion or absorption. Furthermore, inflammation and ulceration of the intestinal mucosa may increase the loss of nutrients from the gut. The most important factor of all, however, is probably anorexia with resultant reduction in food intake; the processes by which parasitic infections impair appetite are poorly understood.

Secondly, malnutrition itself may alter the severity of a parasitic disease (Beisel 1982). The most important means by which this occurs is suppression of immunity. The reduction in resistance to reinfection leads to larger parasite loads. This in turn results in increased severity of disease and further impairment of nutritional status. Thus, since malnutrition and parasitic infections commonly coexist in the same populations in developing countries, a vicious cycle may become established which leads to a progressive deterioration in the health of those communities.

Gastrointestinal parasitic infections are rife in developing countries as a result of both a lack of facilities and behaviour of the population. People squat indiscriminately around the home and in the fields where they work, they commonly defaecate near streams and reservoirs, and use infected human stools as fertilizers in vegetable gardens. Food is often poorly cooked and water is not boiled. Inadequate clothing, particularly footwear, increases exposure to soil-transmitted helminths.

Control and prevention of these infections is most likely to be successful if a holistic approach is adopted with a number of different kinds of interventionist strategies being employed simultaneously (Mata 1982). In the context of the gastrointestinal parasites the most important of these are the provision of effective methods of waste disposal, the installation of safe water supplies and health education to persuade people to use them properly. Unfortunately, these measures are extremely costly and are unlikely to be introduced in many areas in the foreseeable future.

In this chapter, the most important protozoal and helminthic infections of the gastrointestinal tract will be considered. Their epidemiology, pathogenesis, clinical manifestations, methods of diagnosis and treatment will be reviewed briefly. Attention will be paid to the interaction between each organism and the nutritional status of its host. Our understanding of many of these inter-relationships is uncertain and awaits further definitive research (Layrisse & Vargas 1975).

AMOEBIASIS

Amoebiasis occurs throughout the world but is most common in tropical regions. The prevalence of infection in some developing countries approaches 50 per cent, but it is less than 1 per cent in many industrialized countries. The high prevalence rates are probably the result of constant reinfection, the amoebae being transmitted primarily via cysts in contaminated food and water. Following ingestion of cysts, trophozoites excyst in the small intestine. These amoeboid forms divide by binary fission. Trophozoites may be excreted in diarrhoeic stools, while in formed faeces, the parasite shrinks, becomes spherical in shape and secretes a cell wall. The resultant cyst is better able to withstand the rigors of the external environment.

Three organisms have been described, each of which is probably a separate entity, viz *Entamoeba histolytica* (large race > 10 μm diameter), the pathogen; *E. hartmanni* (small race < 10 μm diameter), of doubtful virulence; and *E. histolytica*-like amoeba (low temperature strains), also of doubtful virulence (Diamond 1982). Many earlier studies have failed to distinguish among these amoebae. Furthermore, some strains of *E. histolytica* are virulent, while others are not. These strains cannot be differentiated on morphological grounds, although there are a number of biological and biochemical differences (Sepulveda 1982).

Pathogenesis

The first step in the genesis of amoebic colitis appears to be adhesion of trophozoites to epithelial cells, possibly via a lectin on the parasites' surface. This is followed rapidly by necrosis of epithelial cells, presumably mediated by toxins released by the amoebae. Damaged cells are then phagocytosed by trophozoites (Ravdin & Guerrant 1982). Initially there is little histological evidence of tissue inflammation; subsequent infiltration of inflammatory cells may be in response to secondary bacterial infection. Tissue invasion by amoebae quickly induces specific antibody formation. Cell-mediated immune reactions, however, are not prominent during the early phase of infection, although they may become prominent following successful therapy. Nevertheless, clinical observations of frequent reinfections with *E. histolytica* suggest that little or no protective immunity develops (Trissl 1982).

Clinical features

There is a wide range in the modes of presentation and in the severity of clinical manifestations in that small proportion of patients with amoebic infections who become symptomatic (Adams & MacLeod 1977). The onset is usually gradual over several weeks with the appearance of abdominal discomfort, which may become painful and colicky, and frequent, loose, watery stools containing variable amounts of blood and mucus. Some patients have few constitutional symptoms while others are prostrated. Examination frequently reveals lower abdominal tenderness, and the liver may be slightly enlarged and tender. In severe cases, patients look ill, are febrile, and are dehydrated. Sigmoidoscopy commonly reveals ulcers in the rectal mucosa. The diagnosis is made by finding *E. histolytica* in the stools or in scrapings of rectal mucosa. Amoebic antibodies are found in the serum of 90 per cent or more of patients with invasive amoebiasis.

If left untreated, the symptoms and signs often subside spontaneously after a few weeks or months, but relapses are frequent. A number of complications may supervene; these include fulminant amoebic colitis, perforation with peritonitis, intestinal obstruction or haemorrhage, and extraintestinal spread with abscess formation in the liver, lungs, pericardium and brain.

Effects of amoebic infection on nutritional status

It seems likely that amoebiasis does not usually induce severe malnutrition. Since amoebic infection of the gastrointestinal tract is largely confined to the large bowel, amoebiasis has little effect on absorption of nutrients by the host. Nevertheless, significant loss of endogenous nutrients such as proteins, trace metals and electrolytes in diarrhoeic or dysenteric stools may occur in severely ill patients.

Effects of malnutrition on amoebic infection

The effects of diet on amoebic infection are complex and uncertain. Some reports have indicated a correlation between malnutrition and an increased incidence and greater severity of disease, while others have suggested that malnutrition protects against tissue invasion. Furthermore, it is rarely possible to isolate the role of malnutrition from the effects of other social and environmental factors which may influence the prevalence and severity of amoebiasis (Layrisse & Vargas 1975, Diamond 1982).

For example, Zulus in Durban, South Africa were much more prone to invasive intestinal amoebiasis than were Indians living in the same environment (Elsdon-Dew 1959). It has been proposed that this may be related to their high consumption of maize, either by altering the bowel flora, or as a result of a deficiency of some factors essential for protection. On the other hand, Faust (1958) found a high incidence of amoebic infection but relatively little clinical disease in an improverished population in Colombia. He suggested that the abundance of starch in the intestinal contents may encourage *E. histolytica* to remain in the lumen of the large bowel rather than invade the tissues. Similarly, it was observed that amoebic infection was relatively uncommon among the nomadic Turkana people of Kenya who subsisted principally on milk and were iron deficient. It has been claimed that correction of the iron deficiency increased susceptibility to amoebiasis (Murray et al 1980).

Treatment

Patients with symptomatic amoebiasis may be treated with tinidazole given orally in a daily dose of 30 mg/kg for 3 days.

GIARDIASIS

Giardiasis is found in both temperate and tropical regions, but is more common in the latter, where prevalence rates may reach 30 per cent in young children. Humans are the major reservoir of infection, although there is increasing evidence that a number of animal species such as dogs and beavers may also be involved in some situations. *Giardia lamblia* is transmitted in cyst form both by direct personal contact and in contaminated water (Knight 1980). After cysts are ingested, trophozoites excyst in the upper small intestine. These flagellated organisms divide by binary fission. Some parasites encyst in the gut lumen and are passed in the faeces.

Pathogenesis

Giardia trophozoites appear to roam over the epithelial surface of the small intestine and occasionally adhere directly to the epithelial surface. A variety of mechanisms has been postulated by which the parasites may impair the host's absorption of nutrients (Stevens 1982). These include direct physical blocking by huge numbers of trophozoites covering the villi, the secretion of toxins by the organisms, direct damage to the microvilli by trophozoites, competition with the host for nutrients, impaired absorptive function as a result of mucosal inflammation, and overgrowth of bacteria which compete for nutrients.

Histologically, a variable degree of partial villous atrophy and mononuclear cell infiltration may be seen. *Giardia* trophozoites induce an immune response. This response may be primed by luminal parasites which have been found in contact with lymphocytes, and by occasional trophozoites which migrate between senile epithelial cells and are engulfed by mucosal macrophages. This results in both the production of secretory IgA and cell-mediated immune responses. There may be several consequences of these events. Firstly, significant protective immunity develops. This is suggested by the more frequent development of clinical infection in visitors to endemic areas, and is supported by an experimental study in which a group of prisoners exposed to reinfection were found to be resistant. The importance of humoral immunity is underlined by the frequent association of giardiasis with common variable immunodeficency. Secondly, experimental studies in laboratory animals suggest that immune responses, particularly cell-mediated immune reactions, may be responsible for the pathological changes in the small intestinal mucosa and be necessary for clinical disease (Stevens 1982).

Clinical features

Giardiasis presents a broad clinical spectrum. Many infected persons are asymptomatic, particularly in endemic areas. The acute illness is most marked in those exposed to the organism for the first time. There is frequently a sudden onset of explosive, watery diarrhoea, abdominal distension and discomfort, flatulence, nausea and anorexia. After a week or so, the symptoms either resolve spontaneously or subside into a low-grade, chronic infection with diarrhoea, weight loss and debility which may last for several months. The stools may become greasy and some patients with heavy infections develop a malabsorption syndrome. The diagnosis is made by finding parasites in the stools or in duodenal contents. The relative efficacy of various methods of diagnosis is controversial; much depends upon the skill of the microscopist. Stools should be examined by a direct smear (which will allow detection of both trophozoites and cysts) in the first instance. The recovery of cysts is enhanced by use of a concentration technique (e.g. formol-ether or zinc sulphate); 20–75 per cent of patients have been diagnosed with a single specimen in various series. Excretion of cysts is often intermittent therefore examination of three specimens obtained on alternate days is recommended; this permitted diagnosis in 80–95 per cent of patients. Alternatively, trophozoites can be sought in duodenal contents obtained either by duodenoscopy or by use of an Enterotest[R] capsule in which a nylon string is wound in a gelatine capsule. Trophozoites may also be seen in smears or histological sections of duodenal mucosa obtained at endoscopy or with a Crosby capsule. Finally, a therapeutic trial with an antiparasitic drug may suggest the diagnosis.

Effect of giardiasis on nutritional status

Giardiasis may impair nutrition significantly in some individuals, but in the population at large in endemic areas, it probably has only a minor impact. The infection influences predominantly small bowel function, but there may also be effects on the pancreatic and biliary systems. The net result is malabsorption of fat, carbohydrate and vitamins (Wright 1980, Solomons 1982). The most commonly reported absorptive defect in giardiasis is steatorrhoea. Daily faecal fat excretion in a range of 10–60 g has been reported in 10–60 per cent of subjects in various series. Although doubts have been raised about its significance in this infection, the absorption of D-xylose has been widely regarded as a test for carbohydrate absorption; impaired absorption of this pentose has been reported in 0–55 per cent of patients in a number of series. Digestion of the disaccharides, lactose and sucrose, may be impaired and depression of disaccharidases in small intestinal biopsies has been described. Impaired absorption of vitamin B_{12} has been shown. In general, these parameters return to normal after treatment and eradication of the organisms.

The effects of such malabsorption on growth and development in children are only now being delineated. Treatment of giardiasis in children who were failing to thrive in Melbourne, Australia (where polyparasitism is rare), usually accelerated weight gain (Kay et al 1977). Prophylactic administration of metronidazole to children in a Guatemalan village (where polyparasitism is common) reduced the prevalence of *Giardia* in the stools and resulted in small increases in both height and weight (reviewed in Solomons 1982).

It is probable that gross impairment of nutrition occurs only in that minority of individuals in whom frank malabsorption syndrome develops. In the vast majority of people in endemic areas with subclinical infections, giardiasis may require a minor addition to the overall nutritional requirements of the population.

Effects of malnutrition on giardiasis

Although it could be speculated that malnutrition might increase susceptibility to infection with *Giardia*, little evidence is available to support or refute this view. Theoretically, malnutrition could encourage *Giardia* infection and its effects in a number of ways. These include impairment of immune responses, reduction in the secretion of gastric acid, and bacterial overgrowth in the upper small bowel, all of which are common in protein-energy malnutrition.

Treatment

Symptomatic persons must be treated, as should infected, asymptomatic persons in non-endemic areas. Tinidazole given orally in a single dose of 30 mg/kg is usually satisfactory. Benzoyl metronidazole suspension given in a dose of 50 mg/kg on 3 successive days may be more palatable for young children.

BALANTIDIASIS

Balantidiasis occurs sporadically in many parts of the world. It is not common but is found more frequently in tropical regions. Many mammals are infected but it is probable that pigs and perhaps rats are the major sources of human infections. Occasionally, human to human transmission occurs. Not all the strains recovered from animals are infective to humans. *Balantidium coli* is transmitted by ingestion of cysts in food or water or by direct handling of infected animals. Ciliated trophozoites are released in the bowel.

The parasite usually reproduces by binary fission, but sexual conjugation may sometimes occur. Trophozoites may encyst either within the host or in excreted faeces.

Most infections are asymptomatic and are usually self-limiting. Occasionally, trophozoites invade the mucosa producing an ulcerative colitis with abdominal pain and diarrhoea or dysentery. Tissue invasion is probably facilitated by debility due to intercurrent disease or malnutrition. Since lesions are confined to the large bowel, there is no significant malabsorption in balantidiasis. The diagnosis is made by finding trophozoites or cysts in the stools. Unlike *E. histolytica*, extraintestinal invasion is rare. Treatment with tetracycline 10 mg/kg 3 times daily for several days is usually satisfactory (Zaman 1978).

ISOSPORIASIS

Isosporiasis (intestinal coccidiosis) is an uncommon infection which is found more frequently in the tropics. *Isospora belli* is transmitted by ingestion of food contaminated with cysts. Sporozoites are released from the cysts in the small bowel and invade the mucosa. Here they multiply asexually. Some organisms, however, undergo sexual differentiation. When fertilization of the gametocytes occurs, an oocyst containing two daughter cells develops; in turn sporozoites form within each daughter cells to form a sporocyst. Oocysts in various stages of development are passed in the faeces.

Many infected persons are asymptomatic. Some patients complain of abdominal pain and diarrhoea and develop a low-grade fever; these features usually subside within two or three weeks. In a few of these persons, however, the stools become frankly steatorrhoeic and the duration of the illness is prolonged, resulting in malabsorption syndrome with severe weight loss, and occasionally in death.

The diagnosis is made by finding cysts in the stools. Occasionally, coccidia are seen in a duodenal biopsy. Treatment is difficult but may respond to a prolonged course of pyrimethamine and sulphadiazine (Knight 1978).

A symptomatic or self-limiting infection with mild gastrointestinal disturbances may be produced by *Sarcocystis hominis* or *S. suihominis* (both formerly known as *I. hominis*) after eating uncooked beef or pork, respectively.

HOOKWORM

Hookworm infection is widespread in warm moist regions of the world. Infection is prevalent where sanitation is poor and people walk barefoot. Infective larvae penetrate the intact skin and pass via the bloodstream to the lungs where they enter the alveolar spaces, ascend the airways, and are swallowed. They mature in the small intestine and the adult worms attach themselves to the mucosa by the mouth. Eggs are produced and excreted in the faeces. On the ground, larvae hatch then moult twice to become infective larvae. *Ancylostoma duodenale* may also be acquired by oral ingestion, and it is possible that transmammary transmission may occur.

Humans are the reservoir of the common parasites, *A. duodenale* and *Necator americanus*. A third hookworm, *A. ceylanicum*, which is prevalent in dogs and cats, may also infect man (Miller 1979).

Pathogenesis

Hookworms attach themselves to the intestinal mucosa by sucking several villi into the buccal cavity. Mucosal cells lyse and capillary loops burst; it is probable that blood is both ingested by the worms and escapes around the sides of the parasites. Lysis and haemorrhage are facilitated by secretions of enzymes and an anticoagulant. A mild inflammatory reaction develops around the site of attachment. The worms change their location every 4–6 hours to seek new feeding sites, leaving behind them focal areas of haemorrhage and necrosis. Partial villous atrophy is sometimes seen, but this may reflect intercurrent infection or the effects of malnutrition. Hookworm infection stimulates specific antibody formation, but whether protective immunity with resistance to reinfection occurs is conjectural (Gilman 1982).

Clinical features

Skin penetration by larvae may cause a pruritic, papulovesicular rash, particularly in repeated infections. Migration of larvae through the lungs is usually asymptomatic, but occasionally pulmonary infiltrates with eosinophilia occur. Patients with heavy, acute infections may have abdominal pain and bloody diarrhoea. The majority of persons with light worm loads are asymptomatic. The major manifestations of hookworm disease are iron deficiency anaemia and hypoalbuminaemia with their attendant symptoms and signs.

Diagnosis is made by finding eggs in the faeces. The intensity of infection should be quantitated.

Effects of hookworm infection on nutritional status

The prime factor producing malnutrition in hookworm infection is blood loss. Anorexia as a consequence of this infection may exacerbate the problem. Although impaired absorption of D-xylose, fat and vitamins, as well as flattened jejunal mucosa, have been described in hookworm infection, it is probable that these abnormalities are a consequence of intercurrent infection, tropical sprue, or malnutrition itself. There is no evidence that hookworms themselves have any major nutrient requirements (Layrisse & Vargas 1975, Variyam & Banwell 1982). Whether or not hookworm disease results from hookworm infection depends upon the worm burden (which

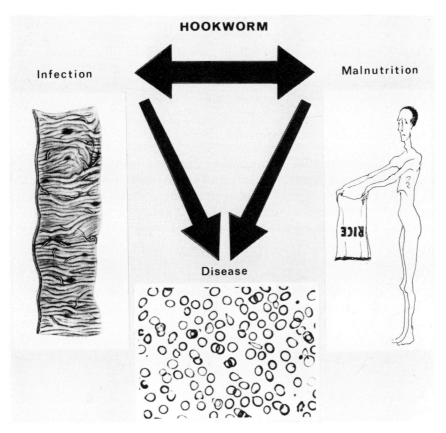

Fig. 6.1 The probability of developing hookworm disease as evidenced by an iron-deficient microcytic anaemia is directly proportional to the worm burden and inversely related to the capacity to replace lost nutrients.

determines blood loss) and nutritional status (which determines the ability to replace lost blood) (Fig. 6.1). For example, in Venezuela, only egg counts of > 5000/g faeces in men were associated with anaemia (Roche & Layrisse 1966).

The average daily blood loss in the faeces produced by hookworms is 0.03 ml/worm for *N. americanus* and 0.2 ml/worm for *A. duodenale* (Roche & Layrisse 1966). When expressed in terms of each 1000 eggs excreted per gram of faeces, the estimated daily blood losses are 2.1 ml and 4.5 ml for these two worms, respectively. Since bleeding generally occurs in the upper bowel, almost 40 per cent of iron lost in the blood may be reabsorbed. In subjects with *Necator* infection and with normal haemoglobin levels, the daily loss of iron in the faeces is approximately 0.7 mg for every 1000 eggs per gram of faeces. If there is a net loss of iron, then an iron-deficient microcytic anaemia develops.

Hypoproteinaemia often accompanies anaemia in patients with heavy hookworm infections. Variable amounts of plasma are lost into the intestinal lumen along with erythrocytes when worms feed. It is probable that a considerable proportion of these leaked proteins can be digested and reabsorbed. Studies of radiolabelled proteins have given contradictory results, and it may be that the hypoproteinaemia is due to an inadequate concurrent protein intake (Variyam & Banwell 1982).

Effect of malnutrition on hookworm infection

Little is known about the effects of malnutrition on hookworm infection in humans. Studies in dogs have shown that malnourished animals had higher *A. caninum* worm burdens. Repletion of protein or iron in humans infected with hookworm, however, did not lead to a reduction in egg output in the stools (Tripathy et al 1971).

Treatment

Patients with symptoms, women and children with egg counts >1000/g faeces, or men with levels >2000/g faeces may be treated with bephenium hydroxynaphthoate 5 g once or mebendazole 100 mg b.d. for 3 days given orally. Iron should be replaced, and when anaemia is very severe, blood transfusion may be necessary.

STRONGYLOIDIASIS

Strongyloidiasis is widespread in warm, moist regions of the world, but it is also found in some temperate areas. The life cycle of *Strongyloides stercoralis* is similar to that of hookworms. Unlike those parasites, however, autoinfection occurs, i.e. rhabditiform larvae released by adult worms develop into infective larvae within the human host and penetrate either the intestinal mucosa or the perianal skin and undergo the usual migration. It is this unusual ability of replicating within man that accounts for the persistence of infection for many years. Humans are the prime reservoir of infection, although dogs and cats may also be infected.

Pathogenesis

A mild inflammatory reaction may be seen around adult worms in the intestinal mucosa. In some patients, there may be partial villous atrophy of the jejunal mucosa. Complete immunity frequently does not develop as indicated by persistent infection. Nevertheless, the infection is contained as the prime manifestations are usually limited to the skin and gastrointestinal tract. In immunosuppressed persons, however, hyperinfection occurs with rapid multiplication and dissemination of worms throughout the body.

Clinical features

Many patients are asymptomatic but others have a variety of cutaneous or gastrointestinal complaints. In larva currens, transient urticarial eruptions migrate in a serpiginous fashion. More commonly, crops of stationary weals appear. Weight loss may develop and patients may complain of diarrhoea, indigestion and lower abdominal pain. In disseminated strongyloidiasis, severe abdominal pain, intestinal obstruction, Gram negative septicaemia, pneumonia and meningitis may supervene.

The diagnosis is made by finding larvae in faeces or duodenal fluid.

Effect of strongyloidiasis on nutritional status

Chronic diarrhoea in strongyloidiasis is associated frequently with weight loss. In heavy infections, a protein-losing enteropathy with marked hypoproteinaemia may result from inflammation of the intestinal mucosa. In some patients, a full-blown malabsorption syndrome develops with steatorrhoea and variable impairment of the absorption of D-xylose, ^{131}I oleic acid, iron, folic acid, and vitamin B_{12} (Milner et al 1965, O'Brien 1975). It is likely that these absorptive defects are more marked if there is concurrent malnutrition (Garcia et al 1977).

Effects of malnutrition on strongyloidiasis

It is well-recognised that overwhelming strongyloidiasis may complicate protein-energy malnutrition (Purtilo et al 1974). Thymolymphatic atrophy with consequent depression of cell-mediated immunity is common in this condition. This permits the widespread dissemination of larvae and participates in the impaired ability to deal with faecal bacteria entering the tissues through intestinal lesions.

Treatment

Infected persons should be treated with thiabendazole 25 mg/kg b.d. orally for 3 days.

ASCARIASIS

Ascariasis is widespread throughout the tropics and subtropics. It is prevalent in areas where sanitation is poor, particularly where human faeces are used as fertiliser. Humans are the reservoir of infection. *Ascaris lumbricoides* is acquired by ingestion of food or soil contaminated with embryonated eggs. Larvae hatch in the small intestine, penetrate the mucosa and pass via the bloodstream to the lungs where they enter the alveolar spaces and ascend the airways; they are swallowed and return to the small bowel where they mature.

Pathogenesis

The pathological responses to migratory larvae are speculative. Adult worms in the intestine rarely cause pathological changes. Radiological studies have shown that most adult worms remain stationary in the jejunum, braced against the intestinal wall. A variety of mechanisms has been postulated by which worms may impair the host's absorption of nutrients (Layrisse & Vargas 1976, Schultz 1982). These include direct competition with the host by consumption of nutrients, interference with absorption due to mucosal lesions, inhibition of the host's digestive enzymes by release of proteolytic agents with antitryptic and antichymotryptic activity, and an increased loss of nutrients as a consequence of increased peristalsis. Immune responses develop during infection, but protective immunity is incomplete. Reinfection occurs rapidly after deworming. It is possible, however, that immune responses may limit the number of parasites in the host at any one time (Pawlowski 1982).

Clinical features

Larval migration through the lungs may be associated with pulmonary infiltrates with eosinophilia, particularly in areas where transmission is seasonal. Most persons with small adult worm loads are either asymptomatic or have ill-defined abdominal discomfort. Occasionally, a bolus of worms may cause intestinal obstruction; this usually happens in young children. Obstructive jaundice has rarely resulted from worms ascending the biliary tree. Ascarids have been found in a number of aberrant sites, but such events occur only in a very small proportion of infected persons.

The diagnosis is made by finding eggs in the faeces. Occasionally, adult worms are passed in the stools.

Effects of ascariasis on nutritional status

Despite intensive investigation, the relationship between ascariasis and malnutrition is controversial and different conclusions have been reached. Stephenson (1980) considered that it is 'clear that in certain communities, *Ascaris* infection is associated with poor growth in malnourished children and that deworming improves growth'. On the other hand, Schultz (1982) is of the view that many studies have been poorly designed, the results have often been contradictory, and many experiments have not been reproducible. He concluded that a 'causal relationship between ascariasis and protein-energy malnurition is not clearly proved'.

One of the earliest clinical studies showed that the excretion of nitrogen in the faeces of infected children fell significantly after deworming. Similarly, impaired absorption of fat and carbohydrate and vitamin A have been claimed in patients with ascariasis. Other studies, however, have failed to support these findings (reviewed in Schultz 1982).

Several community-based studies, in which the effects of deworming on nutrition have been assessed, have appeared recently (Gupta et al 1977, Willett et al 1979, Stephenson et al 1980). Although they have been criticized on a variety of grounds (Schultz, 1982), they all reported that a reduction in worm burden was associated with a small improvement in a number of parameters of nutritional status including height, weight and skinfold thickness.

Effects of malnutrition on ascariasis

These are unknown.

Treatment

All patients should be treated with piperazine citrate 50 mg/kg for 2 days or mebendazole 100 mg twice daily for 3 days given orally.

TRICHURIASIS

Trichuriasis is found in warm, moist regions of the world in areas of poor sanitation. *Trichuris trichiura* is acquired by ingestion of eggs which develop directly into adult worms in the lumen of the bowel and attach to the large bowel mucosa. The vast majority of infected persons are asymptomatic. In heavy infections, diarrhoea, abdominal pain and rectal prolapse may occur. Diagnosis is made by finding eggs in the stools. It is controversial whether blood loss occurs, but one group of investigators estimated that each adult worms sucks 0.005 ml of blood/day. Thus, anaemia is very unlikely to occur as a result of trichuriasis unless patients with marginal nutrition have extremely heavy worm burdens. Such patients may be treated with mebendazole 100 mg given orally twice daily for three days.

SCHISTOSOMIASIS

Schistosoma mansoni is endemic in parts of Africa, the Middle East and Central and South America, while *S. japonicum* is found in parts of Eastern Asia. The infections are prevalent in areas where sanitation is poor and water supplies are inadequate. Larvae (cercariae) penetrate the intact skin when a person comes in contact with infected water. They lose their tails in the process and the resultant schistosomula migrate through the lungs to the portal vessels where they mature. The fertilized female worms release eggs; some embolize to the liver, others are trapped in the intestinal walls, and others escape into the intestinal lumen and are excreted in the faeces. When eggs are deposited in water, larvae (miracidia) hatch and invade certain species of snails; here they multiply and develop into cercariae which are then released into the water.

Pathogenesis

The main factors affecting the severity of disease are the parasite load and the host responses (Warren 1982). The lesions are due, not so much to the egg itself, but to the host reaction to those eggs. Cell-mediated immune processes lead to granuloma formation which may ultimately result in fibrosis. The roles of immune processes in modulating these events and providing resistance to reinfection are controversial.

Clinical features

In acute schistosomiasis, there may be fever, malaise and urticaria. In heavy infections, patients complain of nausea, abdominal pain, vomiting and diarrhoea or dysentery and hepatosplenomegaly may be found; these features usually subside within a few weeks to months. In chronic schistosomiasis, the vast majority of persons have low to moderate worm burdens and are asymptomatic. In heavy infections, hepatomegaly with portal hypertension as indicated by splenomegaly and oesophageal varices may develop; rupture of the latter may cause haematemesis and melaena.

Diagnosis is made by finding eggs in the faeces. The intensity of infection should be quantitated.

Effects of schistosomiasis on nutritional status

Nutritional status appears to be unaffected in the vast majority of patients with schistosomiasis. In those with heavy infections, particularly in people in Egypt where colonic polyposis is common, structural damage to the gastrointestinal mucosa may cause both loss of, and malabsorption of, nutrients (Waslien et al 1973). These include loss of blood (generally < 10 ml per day), albumen, iron, trace elements and vitamins in the faeces. Occasionally, impaired D-xylose absorption, increased faecal fat excretion and glucose intolerance is found (Akpom 1982).

Effects of malnutrition on schistosomiasis

Little information concerning the effects of malnutrition on the severity of schistosomiasis is available, but it is likely that nutritional factors do not have a major role in the natural course of disease (Rocha 1982). For example, no effect could be discerned on faecal egg excretion after giving an enriched diet to malnourished patients (De Witt et al 1964). Concurrent malnutrition, however, may exacerbate some of the clinical features of schistosomiasis, particularly weight loss, anaemia, hypoalbuminaemia, ascites and peripheral oedema. Furthermore, it has been suggested that vegetarian patients may not respond as well as to antischistosomal therapy (Bell 1964).

Treatment

Patients with symptomatic schistosomiasis mansoni or with moderately heavy worm burdens (> 100 eggs/g faeces) may be treated with oxamniquine 15 mg/kg given orally as a single dose. Schistosomiasis japonica may be treated with niridazole given orally 25 mg/kg in divided doses daily for 7 days.

TAENIASIS

Both taeniasis saginata and taeniasis solium are spread widely throughout the world, except that the latter is not found in Oceania. Humans are the only definitive host of these infections. Cattle and pigs are the intermediate hosts for *Taenia saginata* and *T. solium*, respectively. The infection is acquired when meat containing cysts with viable scolices is ingested. The head of the worm attaches to the small intestinal mucosa and develops into an adult worm which may be up to 10 metres long. Segments of worm, which contain the eggs, break off and are passed in the faeces. When ingested by cattle, the larvae hatch, penetrate the mucosa then spread throughout the tissues and develop into cysts. In the case of *T. solium*, however, eggs ingested by humans also behave like those in the intestine of swine.

Pathogenesis

Adult tapeworms in the intestinal lumen usually cause little host reaction and immunity does not develop (Pawlowski & Schultz 1972).

Clinical features

Most patients are asymptomatic, but there may be mild abdominal pain. The most obvious sign of taeniasis is the spontaneous passage of white, motile proglottids. The diagnosis may also be confirmed by finding eggs in the stools.

Nutritional effects

Although it might seem in view of their large size, that tapeworms might utilize significant quantities of nutrients, calculations have suggested that the total amount of worm produced and lost in faeces each year is only about 1 kg (Rees 1967). The absorption of D-xylose and excretion of faecal fat is normal (El-Mawla et al 1966). There is no evidence that malnutrition alters the course of infection.

Treatment

Adults or children more than 6 years of age may be treated with niclosamide 2 g given orally; younger children are given a reduced dose.

REFERENCES

Adams E B, Macleod I N 1977 Invasive amebiasis. I Amebic dysentery and its complications. Medicine (Baltimore) 56: 315–323
Akpom C A 1982 Schistosomiasis: nutritional implications. Reviews of Infectious Diseases 4: 776–782
Beisel W R 1982 Synergism and antagonism of parasitic diseases and malnutrition. Reviews of Infectious Diseases 4: 746–750
Bell D R 1964 Diet and therapy in bilharzia. Lancet i: 643–644
De Witt W B, Oliver-Gonzales J, Medina E 1964 Effects of improving the nutrition of malnourished people infected with Schistosoma mansoni. American Journal of Tropical Medicine and Hygiene 13: 25–35
Diamond L S 1982 Amebiasis: nutritional implications. Reviews of Infectious Diseases 4: 843–850
El-Mawla N G, Abdallah A, Galil N 1966 Studies on the malabsorption syndrome among Egyptians (5) Faecal fat and D-xylose tests in patients with ascariasis and taeniasis. Journal of the Egyptian Medical Association 49: 473–476
Elsdon-Dew R 1959 Factors influencing the pathogenicity of Entamoeba histolytica In: Proceedings of the World Congress of Gastroenterology and the fifty-ninth annual meeting of the American Gastroenterological Association. Williams & Wilkins, Baltimore, vol 2, p 770–773
Faust E C 1958 Parasitological surveys in Cali, Departomento de Valle, Colombia I Incidence and morphological characteristics of strains of Entamoeba histolytica. American Journal of Tropical Medicine and Hygiene 7: 4–15
Garcia F T, Seesions J T, Strum W B, Schweistris E, Tripathy K, Bolanos O et al 1977 Intestinal function and morphology in strongyloidiasis. American Journal of Tropical Medicine and Hygiene 26: 859–865
Gilman R H 1982 Hookworm disease: host-pathogen biology. Reviews of Infectious Diseases 4: 824–829
Gupta M C, Mithal S, Arora K L, Tandon B N 1977 Effect of periodic deworming on nutritional status of Ascaris-infested preschool children receiving supplementary food. Lancet ii: 108–110
Kay R, Barnes G L, Townley R R W 1977 Giardia lamblia infestation in 154 children. Australian Paediatric Journal 13: 98–104
Keusch G T, Migasena P 1982 Biological implications of poly-parasitism. Reviews of Infectious Diseases 4: 880–882
Knight R 1978 Giardiasis, isosporiasis and balantidiasis. Clinics in Gastroenterology 7: 31–47
Knight R 1980 Epidemiology and transmission of giardiasis. Transactions of the Royal Society of Tropical Medicine and Hygiene 74: 433–436
Layrisse M, Vargas A 1975 Nutrition and intestinal parasitic infection. Progress in Food and Nutrition Science 1: 645–667
Mata L 1982 Sociocultural factors in the control and prevention of parasitic diseases. Reviews of Infectious Diseases 4: 871–879
Miller T A 1979 Hookworm infection in man. Advances in Parasitology. 17: 315–384
Milner P F, Irvine R A, Barton C J, Bras G, Richards R 1965 Intestinal malabsorption in Strongyloides stercoralis infestation. Gut 6: 574–581
Murray M J, Murray A B, Murray C J 1980 The salutary effect of milk on amoebiasis and its reversal by iron. British Medical Journal 280: 1351–1352

O'Brien W 1975 Intestinal malabsorption in acute infection with *Strongyloides stercoralis*. Transactions of the Royal Society of Tropical Medicine and Hygiene 69: 69–77

Pawlowski Z S 1982 Ascariasis: host-pathogen biology. Reviews of Infectious Diseases 4: 806–814

Pawlowski A, Schultz M G 1972 Taeniasis and cysticercosis (*Taenia saginata*). Advances in Parasitology 10: 269–343

Purtilo D T, Meyers W M, Connor D H 1974 Fatal strongyloidiasis in immunosuppressed patients. American Journal of Medicine 56: 488–493

Ravdin J I, Guerrant R L 1982 A review of the parasite cellular mechanisms involved in the pathogenesis of amoebiasis. Reviews of Infectious Diseases 4: 1185–1207

Rees G 1967 Pathogenesis of adult cestodes. Helminthological Abstracts 36: 1–23

Rocha H 1982 Discussion : schistosomiasis and malnutrition. Reviews of Infectious Diseases 4: 783–784

Roche M, Layrisse M 1966 Nature and causes of 'hookworm anemia' American Journal of Tropical Medicine and Hygiene 15: 1029–1102

Rosenberg I H, Bowman B B 1982 Intestinal physiology and parasitic diseases. Reviews of Infectious Diseases 4: 763–767

Schultz M G 1982 Ascariasis: nutritional implications. Reviews of Infectious Diseases 4: 815–819

Sepulveda B 1982 Amebiasis: host-pathogen biology. Reviews of Infectious Diseases 4: 1247–1253

Solomons N W 1982 Giardiasis: nutritional implications. Reviews of Infectious Diseases 4: 859–869

Stephenson L S 1980 The contribution of *Ascaris lumbricoides* to malnutrition in children. Parasitology 81: 221–233

Stevens D P 1982 Giardiasis: host-pathogen biology. Reviews of Infectious Diseases 4: 851–858

Tomkins A M 1979 The roles of intestinal parasites in diarrhoea and malnutrition. Tropical Doctor 9: 21–24

Tripathy K, Garcia F T, Lotero H 1971 Effect of nutritional repletion on human hookworm infection. American Journal of Tropical Medicine and Hygiene 20: 219–223

Trissl D 1982 Immunology of *Entamoeba histolytica* in human and animal hosts. Reviews of Infectious Diseases 4: 1154–1184

Variyam E P, Banwell J G 1982 Hookworm disease: nutritional implications. Reviews of Infectious Diseases 4: 830–835

Warren K S 1982 Schistosomiasis: host-pathogen biology. Reviews of Infectious Diseases 4: 771–775

Waslien C I, Farid Z, Darby W J 1973 The malnutrition of parasitism in Egypt. Southern Medical Journal 66: 47–50

Willett W C, Kilama W L, Kihamia C M 1979 *Ascaris* and growth rates: a randomized trial of treatment. American Journal of Public Health 69: 987–991

Wright S C 1980 Giardiasis and malabsorption. Transactions of the Royal Society of Tropical Medicine and Hygiene 74: 436–437

Zaman V 1978 *Balantidium coli*. In: J P Kreier (ed) Parasitic protozoa, vol II. Academic Press, New York, p 633–653

Lactose intolerance

The mammary gland of placental animals is the only known source of naturally occurring disaccharide lactose. It is absent from the milk of the California Sea Lion (Kretchmer & Sunshine 1967) and human milk contains the highest concentration of the disaccharide (7–7.5 g/100 ml). It is the only source of carbohydrate in the diet of newborn humans.

The enzyme, lactase, is situated in the brush border of the mucosal lining of the gastrointestinal tract. Enzyme activity increases from the proximal to the distal duodenum (Welsh et al 1966) with peak activity occurring in the jejunum or proximal ileum. Levels in the ileum are low (Auricchio et al 1965).

β-Glycosidases (lactase and cellobiase) develop late in intrauterine life and reach maximum values only at the end of normal gestation (Auricchio et al 1965). Premature infants are therefore naturally lactose malabsorbers, but after birth feeding induces a rapid increase in enzyme activity, and by 1 to 2 weeks of age, it reaches that of full-term babies (Jarrett & Holman 1966, Boellner et al 1965). The level of enzyme activity attained is probably insufficient to hydrolyse the large lactose load in milk fed to premature and full-term babies even if the entire small intestine were assumed to be acting maximally 24 hours a day (Auricchio et al 1965). There is evidence indicating that this is probably so, as significant amounts of reducing substances, including glucose, galactose and lactose, have been detected in the stools of infants who were breast-fed or fed modified cow's-milk formula (Davidson & Mullinger 1970) who have no symptoms and continue to gain weight normally.

The pattern of development of intestinal lactase activity as demonstrated in mammals, e.g. the rat, pig, dog and rabbit (Plimmer 1906, Doell & Kretchmer 1962) after infancy is such that its activity declines at approximately the weaning period to reach very low levels in adults. This decline has also been demonstrated in children in many countries. The age at which it occurs has been reported as 42 months in Ugandan children (Cook 1967), 1–2 years in children in institutions and over 2 years in village Thai children (Keusch et al 1965) and 2–4 years in Nigerian children (Kretchmer et al 1971).

The degree of this decline, and so the prevalence of lactose malabsorption, rises with age. For example, in full-blooded Pima Indian children of Arizona, 40 per cent were malabsorbers at the age of 3–4 years, 71 per cent at age 4–5 years and 92 per cent at age 5–7 years; all children studied over the age of 8 years were lactose malabsorbers (Johnson et al 1977).

Most racial groups in the world follow this mammalian pattern whereby 80–100 per cent of the adult population are lactose malabsorbers (Kretchmer 1977).

There are some racial groups in which this decline does not occur and their adults are lactose absorbers. Examples of these are North Americans (Bayless & Rosensweig 1966), Northern Europeans (Jussila 1969), Caucasians, the Fulani in Nigeria (Kretchmer et al 1971) and the Tussis in Uganda (Cook & Kajubi 1966).

DIAGNOSIS OF LACTOSE INTOLERANCE

Loading tests

Intestinal lactase deficiency can be demonstrated by performing an oral lactose loading test; 2 g/kg body weight of lactose to a maximum of 50 g is administered to an individual after an overnight fast. Capillary blood, so as to minimize false positive results, i.e. flat curves (Welsh et al 1967, Welsh 1970, McGill & Newcomer 1967), is collected at 0, 15, 30, 60 and 90 minutes after ingestion of lactose. A rise of less than 20 mg/100 ml of blood glucose above fasting levels in any of the blood specimens plus the occurrence of symptoms during the 24 hours after the loading dose constitutes presumptive evidence of lactose intolerance. Individuals in whom a 'flat' curve is obtained but who do not have symptoms for 24 hours after the test are malabsorbers. This is particularly common in children.

False negative tests may be obtained if there is delayed gastric emptying, if venous rather than capillary blood is used for the glucose estimation, and if the patient is diabetic. To rule out intestinal malabsorption due to inflammatory or other gut diseases, a glucose–galactose (25 g or 1 g/kg body weight for each monosaccharide) tolerance test should be carried out. A normal rise (i.e. over 20 mg/100 ml of blood glucose) indicates that the individual is able to absorb the constituent monosaccharides of lactose.

Welsh (1970) concluded that there were less than 1 per cent false tests in lactose tolerant subjects and 7 per cent in intolerant individuals using capillary blood for glucose estimations.

Intestinal enzyme activity

Lactase activity can be determined by biochemical assay of intestinal biopsy specimens for the enzyme (Dahlqvist 1964). It is important, at the same time, to describe the morphology of the intestinal mucosa in the biopsy specimen; this will be normal in those subjects in whom lactase deficiency is not secondary to intestinal disease. Good correlation has been found between flat lactose tolerance tests and intestinal lactase activity (Cook & Kajubi 1966, Welsh 1970).

Breath tests

The estimation of breath hydrogen concentration after a lactose load is a non-invasive method which can now be used to detect lactose malabsorption. On reaching the colon, any unabsorbed lactose is fermented by bacterial activity liberating various gases, including hydrogen. These gases enter the portal circulation and are expired in the breath (Bond & Levitt 1976a). Peak hydrogen levels can be detected in the breath of lactose intolerant individuals within $2\frac{1}{2}$ to 3 hours after taking 50 g of lactose or a volume of milk containing the same weight of lactose. This is not so in lactose intolerant individuals (Calloway et al 1969). Nose et al (1979) applied the method to investigate lactose malabsorption in children and adults. They recommended a loading dose of 1 g/kg of lactose which will produce a measurable increase of breath hydrogen greater than 0.05 ml/min/m^2.

Lactose-barium meal

Barium meal studies, incorporating lactose, show a characteristic picture of dilution of the contrast medium, dilatation of the small bowel and rapid intestinal transit. This is a useful adjunct in the diagnosis of lactose intolerance (Neale 1968) particularly when the result of a lactose tolerance test is doubtful and biopsy is either not possible or not indicated.

Screening tests on stools

Stool acidity resulting from lactose fermentation and the presence of reducing substances in stools due to unabsorbed lactose, are useful screening tests for lactose intolerance. Reducing substances can easily be detected using commercially available 'Clinitest' tablets with fresh specimens of stools (Kerry & Anderson 1964).

A high percentage of the stools of normal neonates and infants breast-fed or receiving artificial milk with 7 per cent lactose may give a positive test for reducing substances (Davidson & Mullinger 1970) and the stools of infants with infective gastroenteritis may have a low pH. The results of these tests should therefore be interpreted with caution.

If the concentration of reducing substances in stools is above 0.25 per cent and/or the pH is less than 6, infants with diarrhoea can be considered to have lactose malabsorption (Lifshitz et al 1971).

PATHOPYHSIOLOGY OF LACTOSE INTOLERANCE

After a meal containing lactose, the rate of gastric emptying is increased in individuals with lactase deficiency (Pirk & Skala 1972, Welsh & Hall 1977). One might speculate that rapid emptying could play a role in the development of symptoms since, for any given load, the small intestine should deal more easily with sugar that empties slowly as a steady stimulus rather than with a large single bolus (Phillips 1981).

In the small intestine, the residual intestinal lactase hydrolyses a portion of the lactose ingested so producing glucose and galactose. The rise in blood glucose which follows a lactose tolerance test reflects the amount of the residual enzymatic activity. Bond & Levitt (1976b) showed that while 0.9–8 per cent of a 12.5 g dose of lactose was recovered from the ileum of lactose absorbers, 42 to 75 per cent was recoverable in individuals with hypolactasia.

Small amounts of lactose diffuse across the intestinal mucosa into the blood stream, and are excreted in the urine. In the rabbit, the amount of lactose which enters the circulation depends on its concentration in the intestinal lumen (Sterk & Kretchmer 1964). This finding is not specific to individuals with lactose malabsorption as it also occurs in other conditions such as infection, hyperthyroidism and various small bowel diseases (Alpers & Isselbacher 1970).

The retention of lactose in the lumen of the small intestine in lactose malabsorbers provides an osmotic force for water and sodium to be drawn into the lumen. Thus, the volume of fluid within the intestinal lumen increases (Launiala 1968, Christopher & Bayless 1971, quoted by Phillips 1981). Studies also indicate that the presence of lactose in the small intestine decreases the transit time of its contents (Debongnie et al 1979).

In the large intestine, lactose is fermented by colonic bacteria to produce short-chain fatty acids, carbon dioxide and hydrogen. The lactose and organic acids increase the osmolality of the bowel contents; however, the ability of the intestine to absorb gases (Bond & Levitt 1976b), organic ions (Ruppin et al 1980), sodium, chloride and water remains unimpaired. Analysis of the fluid entering the colon indicates that about two-thirds of the osmotic load consists of endogenous electrolyte. Bond and Levitt's (1976b) studies suggest that the colonic absorption of bacterially produced organic acids may be the mechanism whereby the normal, formed stool is produced despite the failure of the small bowel to absorb material with an appreciable osmotic activity. They suggest that lessening of diarrhoea which often occurs in lactase deficient individuals after long-term consumption of milk, may be explained by the induction of a lactose-fermenting flora better able to metabolize the sugar. The occurrence of diarrhoea in a susceptible subject after a lactose load might depend, therefore, on a balance being struck on each occasion between the absorptive properties of the colon which will minimise symptoms and important, but poorly documented, additional factors in any individual which may include the nature of the colonic flora and transit time of material through the colon (Phillips 1981).

Absorbed short-chain fatty acids produced by the metabolism of disaccharides by colonic bacteria provide 16 per cent of the total energy requirements of the porcupine (Johnson & McBee 1967) and 4.7 per cent of those of the rat (Young et al 1970). Organic anions produced in this way may also be a source of energy in humans.

PATTERNS OF LACTOSE INTOLERANCE

Congenital lactase deficiency

This was first described by Holzel et al (1959), and later by Lifshitz (1966) and Levin and his colleagues (1970).

Watery diarrhoea starts soon after the beginning of breast or cow's milk feeding. The babies, however, have a good appetite, are lively and there is no vomiting. Dehydration and acidosis develop, but these babies can survive for months in this state. Growth is retarded and malnutrition develops.

The response to elimination of lactose from the diet is prompt. Diarrhoea stops immediately and rapid growth takes place.

If feeding of lactose is prolonged before diagnosis, intestinal villous atrophy may occur and be accompanied by impaired intestinal absorption. These changes are reversible once lactose feeds are stopped. The condition is inherited as an autosomal recessive gene (Savilahti et al 1983).

Secondary lactose intolerance

Following diseases of the gastrointestinal tract, damage to the epithelium of the intestinal mucosa may lead to lactose malabsorption. Examples of such diseases are gastroenteritis (Sunshine & Kretchmer 1964, Wharton et al 1968), malnutrition (Bowie et al 1965), coeliac disease (Lubos et al 1967), viral hepatitis (Chalfin & Holt 1967) and tropical sprue (Gray et al 1968). Rotavirus and Norwalk agent enteral infection (Gall 1980, Kapikian 1976), *Giardia lamblia* infestations, and immunological deficiencies are other examples (Dubois et al 1970).

Rotaviruses seems to be a major cause of diarrhoea and carbohydrate intolerance in infancy. It has been postulated that intestinal lactase is the receptor and uncoating enzyme for these enteric viruses (Holmes et al 1976). Before diarrhoea occurs, the virus must infect gut epithelium rich in lactase. This hypothesis is consistent with the high prevalence of lactose intolerance in gastroenteritis in infancy (Lifshitz Coello — Ramirez and Contreras — Guitierrez 1971).

Certain systemic disorders may be accompanied by lactose intolerance. For example in the newborn, hypoxia may be a factor in precipitating lactose intolerance (Akesode et al 1973, Book et al 1976) due to a decreased

(Na^+-K^+) adenosine triphosphatase activity in the intestinal mucosa (Lifshitz et al 1974). Disaccharide intolerance may also lead to severe complications such as monosaccharide intolerance and necrotizing enterocolitis (Akesode et al 1973, Book et al 1976, Tejani et al 1979). The recovery of premature infants may be hindered by carbohydrate intolerance which sometimes follows neonatal asphyxia (Tejani et al 1979).

Intestinal lactase deficiency in malnourished children may persist for up to a year after recovery (Bowie et al 1967). In Indian children with malnutrition, lactase deficiency was found to be reversed on recovery (Chandra et al 1968). It can be impossible to decide whether the lactase deficiency is due to mucosal damage or genetic in origin unless lactose tolerance tests had been performed before the onset of malnutrition.

Late-onset hypolactasia

Due to the normal decline of intestinal lactase activity after weaning, adults in the majority of the world's populations have been found to be unable to digest lactose. This is now recognized as the 'normal' state after childhood.

Evidence has been adduced to indicate that communities with a large population of adult lactose absorbers have a very long history of dairying and this are thought to have acquired the ability to digest lactose in later life. 'Plotting of known percentage of tolerance and intolerance on a map of the world areas of milking and non-milking as of 1500 A.D. would provide one interesting conclusion: to date not a single human group with a low incidence of intolerance (less than 30 per cent of the population sampled) has been discovered that is native to the traditional areas of non-milking' (Simoons 1973). It must be recognized that this ability to digest lactose represents a deviation from the typical mammalian pattern.

The populations studied so far can be divided into three groups (Fig. 7.1) (Kretchmer 1977).

1. Those with a high incidence of lactose malabsorbers (80%). These are those who live in a classical non-milking zone and cannot digest lactose. This group will include all aboriginal peoples of the Americas (Johnson et al 1977, 1978) and Australia (Brand et al 1983), East Asians, and many African peoples, for example the Yorubas of Nigeria (Kretchmer et al 1971), and the Bantus of East Africa (Cook & Kajubi 1966).

2. Those with a low incidence of lactose malabsorbers (10–30 per cent). They live in a milking zone and can digest lactose. This group includes Northern Europeans, for example Finns (Jussila 1969), Danes (Gudmand-Hoyer & Jarnum 1969), the pastoralist Fulani of Nigeria (Kretchmer et al 1971) and the Tussis of Uganda (Cook & Kajubi 1966).

3. Those with an incidence of lactose malabsorption intermediate between 1 and 2 (i.e. 40–70 per cent). These people live in a milking zone and cannot digest lactose. This group includes Hausas of Northern Nigeria (Kretchmer et al 1971), American Blacks (Bayless & Rosensweig 1966) and

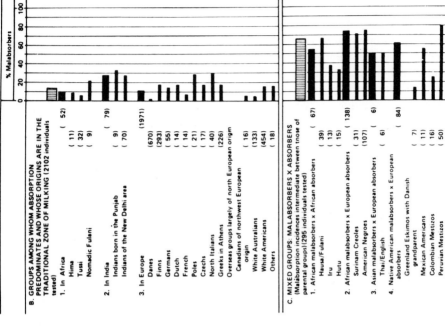

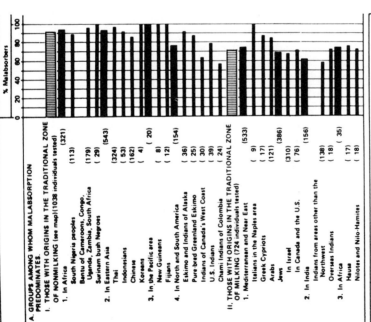

Fig. 7.1 Differences in lactose malabsorption among the world's peoples (adults). (Taken from Johnson J D et al 1974 Advances in Paediatrics 21: 197, by permission of the Editor.)

Mediterranean and Middle Eastern peoples. These people were originally pure lactose malabsorbers but, due to inbreeding with the native lactose absorbers, many have inherited the lactose digesting gene.

Genetic studies on the ability to digest lactose (the abnormal state) in mixed marriages among Nigerians (Ransome-Kuti et al 1975), and the Pima Indians of Arizona (Johnson et al 1977) indicate that it is inherited as an autosomal dominant gene.

CLINICAL FEATURES OF LACTOSE INTOLERANCE

These stem from the action of the unabsorbed lactose on intestinal motility which is increased (Debongnie et al 1979) giving rise to borborygmi. The intestinal bacterial flora digests the unabsorbed lactose thus releasing gases which cause flatus and abdominal distension. The increased volume of intestinal intraluminal contents which is caused by the osmotic action of the unabsorbed lactose (Christopher & Bayless 1971) and its bacterial degradation products (Torres-Pinedo et al 1966) causes diarrhoea.

Premature and newborn babies

Premature babies are able to ingest breast or cow's milk formula without symptoms even if they are lactase deficient (Maclean & Fink 1981). However, the colonic microflora of breast-fed infants differs substantially from that of bottle-fed infants (Bullen et al 1977). The faecal flora of predominantly lactose fermenters, as opposed to putrefactive bacteria, may favour intestinal colonization with organisms that tend to be less pathogenic to the infant (Maclean & Fink 1981).

In populations with a high prevalence of adult hypolactasia, an early fall of intestinal lactase activity, within the first 6 to 12 weeks of life, has been reported in normal newborn babies (Cook 1967). King (1972) has reported that in Zambia, an area with a high rate of adult hypolactasia (Cook et al 1973), diarrhoea is common during the early breast-feeding period and usually ceases by the time of weaning.

Hoskova et al (1980) reported severe vomiting, lactosuria, amino-aciduria and elevated serum transaminases in a 3-week-old breast-fed infant who responded to a milk-free diet. Although a lactose tolerance test was not done at the onset of the episode, because of the child's serious condition, biochemical lactose tolerance was normal at the age of 5 months and the infant tolerated milk feeds at the age of 6 months. This may represent a situation in which there was a delay in the maturation of intestinal lactase.

Children

Even when lactose malabsorption is demonstrated by means of lactose tolerance tests, symptoms are uncommon in children within 24 hours of the test. The available data suggest symptoms appear after a lactose tolerance test with increasing frequency as age increases, and that there is a relationship between decreasing lactase activity, incomplete lactose digestion and symptoms with increasing age (Paige 1981). There seem to be a sharp rise in the incidence of symptoms after the age of 8 years in American children (Paige 1981). Data from Nigeria (Olatunbosun & Adadevoh 1972), Singapore (Bolin et al 1970) and Arizona (Johnson et al 1977) indicate that 100% of children at about the same age were lactose malabsorbers as shown by lactose tolerance tests.

When children were classified as milk drinkers if they consumed 50 per cent or more by weight of a 240 ml (8 ounce) glass of milk per 24 hours, Bayless & Paige (1979) (quoted in Paige 1981) found that, below the age of 8 years, approximately 10 per cent of American black children failed to meet these criteria and were designated non-milk drinkers. At 8 years of age, over 20 per cent of the observed children were classified as non-milk drinkers. The studies of Garza & Scrimshaw (1976) also support the view that declining levels of lactase may have little or no clinical consequence in populations of healthy children below 8 years of age.

Symptoms, mainly flatulence and abdominal distension, experienced by lactose intolerant children after drinking milk are usually mild. The condition has, however, been demonstrated to be a probable cause of recurrent abdominal pain which was relieved on withdrawal of lactose from the diet (Barr et al 1979, Liebman 1979).

The risk of causing symptoms related to lactose intolerance has led to questioning the use of milk in nutritional supplementation programmes in areas with a high prevalence of lactose malabsorption, particularly in rural areas where the prevalence of gastrointestinal symptoms is high. Lisker et al (1980) partly attributed the high rate of milk intolerance in rural Mexican children to gastrointestinal infections. Australian Aboriginal children suspected to have intestinal hypolactasia when fed normal milk were found to excrete more fat and perhaps other nutrients including fat-soluble vitamins in the stool than those who were fed hydrolysed milk; stool frequency as well as stool wet weight were similar on both regimes (Brand & Mitchell 1980). Studies in Bangladesh led Brown (1981) to conclude that, 'it appears that milk can be tolerated and utilized well by young lactose malabsorbers when it is provided in relatively low doses and with additional food sources'. He suggested that, 'milk not be delivered as a single source of energy in a supplemented feeding programme in the tropics. Instead, it should be mixed with the traditionally consumed weaning and children's foods to bolster their protein and energy density. The milk should be introduced into the diet slowly and faecal excretion patterns should be monitored to determine how well the supplement is absorbed. Used in this way, milk can provide an important nutritional supplement even in settings where lactose malabsorption is common'. Brown found a strong correlation between mean daily faecal wet weight and faecal loss of energy and carbohydrate. If faecal weight increases excessively on a diet containing lactose, increased energy losses will be likely. However, if faecal excretion is not increased then normal nutrient absorption can be assumed. This correlation is potentially useful to auxiliaries supervizing feeding programmes (Brown 1981).

Adults

Many lactose malabsorbers either do not give a history of symptoms following drinking milk, or more commonly do not recognize the relationship of symptoms to milk ingested. Most of these people limit their intake of milk to small quantities, usually with tea, and so do not have symptoms; others use milk for its laxative effect (Welsh 1970). The occurrence of symptoms appears to depend on the ingestion of threshold quantities of lactose. It is common for milk intolerance to be identified for the first time when large amounts of milk are given in therapeutic diets and the threshold exceeded (Dunphy et al 1965). Three-quarters of lactose intolerant adults studied by Bedine & Bayless (1973) developed symptoms with the amount of lactose found in 8 ounces of milk. Ten of the 15 subjects gave a history of awareness of milk intolerance. When the investigators interviewed persons with low lactase levels, some were aware of abdominal cramps, bloating, flatulence and even diarrhoea after drinking one glass of milk, while some needed to drink three or four glasses of milk at one sitting to have symptoms. Others had no symptoms.

Among the Bantus of Uganda, a population of lactose malabsorbers, no correlation was found between milk intake and intestinal lactase activity. Five of the 12 Bantus studied drank 600 ml of milk apparently without symptoms whereas 4 of the 6 Hamitic subjects, who were lactose absorbers, drank 600 ml or less daily (Cook & Dahlqvist 1968, Cook, undated manuscript).

The fact that lactose malabsorbers can tolerate large quantities of milk without symptoms probably means that an adaptive process has taken place. Only 1 of the 11 lactose intolerant persons investigated by Mitchell et al (1975) was aware of milk intolerance and admitted that he drank no milk because of this awareness.

In Iran, Sabre & Kabrashi (1979) noted a high rate of rejection of milk by lactose-intolerant school children at the start of a milk supplementation programme. As the programme was continued, the initial rates of rejection of milk fell.

In 10 lactose deficient adults given more than 1 litre of milk daily for 6 to 14 months, jejunal lactase remained low after this period although after an initial adjustment period, the patients tolerated their considerable milk intake remarkably well (Gilat et al 1972).

Lactose intolerant medical students in Lagos were fed increasing amounts of lactose over a period of 6 months until they were able to take 50 g a day without symptoms. Repeat lactose tolerance test at the end of the period showed that they were still malabsorbers (Kretchmer 1977). Keusch et al 1969 demonstrated that feeding 25 g of lactose twice a day for an average of 26 days to 50 healthy adult Thais did not induce increased intestinal lactase activity.

MANAGEMENT OF LACTOSE MALABSORPTION

Newborns with congenital hypolactasia cease to have diarrhoea as soon as a lactose-free diet is instituted. Rapid weight gain soon follows.

Institution of lactose-free diets in premature babies on the basis of tests indicating lactose malabsorption, is not justified unless symptoms are present. The replacement of cow's milk formula or breast milk with lactose-free formulas in these babies may not be without dangers since it has been shown that lactose in milk normally facilitates the absorption of calcium in experimental animals, even in those with low intestinal lactase levels (Leichter & Tolensky 1975). A preliminary report suggests that this is true in the human infant as well (Zeigler & Fomon 1980, quoted by Maclean & Fink 1981).

Similarly, newborns and infants, known to have significant amounts of reducing substances, including lactose, in their stools during breast and formula feeding but without symptoms and weight loss, should not be placed on lactose-free milk (Davidson & Mullinger 1970).

Secondary lactose intolerance often develops in infants following gastroenteritis. In breast-feeding infants, although breast milk contains a high concentration of lactose, breast feeding should be continued. Their tolerance of breast milk may be due to the presence of substances such as the large amount of Bifidus factor (Gyorgy 1953). Breast milk also has other immunological qualities that may help in the treatment of the diarrhoea. However, if the diarrhoea persists on breast milk, the use of milk containing other sugars should be substituted for the duration of the episode.

In babies fed cow's milk, this should be stopped in the initial phase of the diarrhoea, and a diet containing sucrose can be substituted. This reduces the severity and duration of the diarrhoea (Dagan et al 1980). The sucrose-containing diet should be continued for two to three weeks to allow regeneration of the damaged intestinal mucosal lining (Hyams et al 1981). This diet also promotes more weight gain than one containing lactose even after recovery from diarrhoea (Strickland et al 1979).

In lactose intolerant children, elimination of lactose from the diet reduces the occurrence of recurrent abdominal pain and this increases in frequency when lactose is reintroduced (Barr et al 1979, Watkins 1981). Malnourished children with kwashiorkor are reported to benefit from a milk diet even when it causes some diarrhoea (Bowie 1975). The dangers of severe dehydration and circulatory changes must be weighed against the benefits derived from drinking milk when pursuing this course. Should diarrhoea prove a greater threat, it is wise to substitute a lactose-free diet for milk

(Prinsloo et al 1969, Wharton et al 1968). Such a diet can be devised so that it is based on locally available foodstuffs in communities where kwashiorkor is common. After treatment, lactase deficiency persists longer than do deficiencies of other small intestinal disaccharidases (Cook & Lee 1966, Bowie et al 1967).

Adolescents and adults do not need to take milk or its products for nutritional reasons. Milk should be avoided at this age if it causes symptoms. When the limits of intestinal lactase are exceeded in these individuals, symptoms develop which are usually not attributed to milk drinking by them. Lactase intolerant adults and adolescents either avoid milk or regularly consume quantities which do not produce symptoms. If they develop symptoms yet enjoy drinking milk, their symptoms are either ignored or tolerated.

Patients with ulcerative colitis (Tandon et al 1971), cystic fibrosis (Antonowicz et al 1968), following intestinal resection and some adults with the irritable colon syndrome (Weser et al 1965, McMichael et al 1965) with lactose intolerance have had their symptoms relieved after the removal of milk from their diets.

Treating peptic ulcers in lactose malabsorbers with milk may not be advisable, especially if milk is taken far in excess of the ability of their intestinal lactase hydrolytic activity to cope with it. Seven out of eight patients with peptic ulcer who developed symptoms after the institution of a high-milk diet were found to be lactase deficient; three of them were black (Welsh 1970).

Hydrolysed milks have been developed which are well tolerated by lactase deficient individuals (Dahlqvist 1977, Paige et al 1975). In most older lactose malabsorbing children, it seems that incomplete lactose digestion can be significantly improved by substituting a lactose-hydrolysed milk for cow's milk (Paige et al 1975). This has recently been shown in rural children who have a high incidence of inadequate nutrition, diarrhoea and intestinal parasites (Lisker et al 1980).

LACTOSE INTOLERANCE IN PERSPECTIVE

With the intensive study of lactose malabsorption during the past 20 years, its true significance is beginning to emerge. In predominantly lactose malabsorbing communities, it is important for the inhabitants to recognize that ingestion of large quantities of milk and its products by older children and adults may cause gastrointestinal symptoms. In this way unnecessary investigations and treatments can be prevented. Where there is no indigenous milk industry, the intensive promotion of milk-drinking in lactose malabsorbing communities may cause serious disadvantages in terms of morbidity in the population. This should be recognized and discouraged by the relevant health authorities.

However, where there is an established dairy industry and large quantities of milk are generally available, lactose malabsorbers may drink milk with no ill effect, perhaps because of individual intestinal adaptation. For example, the Bantus of South Africa, a lactose malabsorbing racial group consume milk every day in quantities about the same as their Caucasian counterparts without symptoms (Jersky & Kinsley 1967). The same situation exists among many American blacks.

In 1972, the Protein Advisory Group of the United Nations issued a statement indicating that it would be highly inappropriate, on the basis of available evidence, to discourage programmes aimed to improve milk supplies and to increase milk consumption among children because of the risk of milk intolerance. Since then, it has become clear that in children under the age of 8 years (which includes preschool children), lactose malabsorption is of little practical importance. Above this age, and especially in children in the rural areas with intestinal parasite infection (Lisker et al 1980), the increasing importance of symptoms with increasing age must be recognized. Inter-racial and intertribal marriages are slowly spreading the lactose-absorbing gene to non-lactose absorbing communities. Dairying is also slowly gaining ground in many countries. There may come a time when this gene may predominate in most or all parts of the world and man may truly become a lactose absorbing mammal.

REFERENCES

Akesode F, Lifshitz F, Hoffman M 1973 Transient monosaccharide intolerance in a newborn infant. Pediatrics 51: 891–97
Alpers D H, Isselbacher K J 1970 Disaccharidase deficiency. Advances in Metabolic Disorders 4: 75–122
Antonowicz I, Reddy V, Khaw K T, Shwachman H 1968 Lactase deficiency in patients with cystic fibrosis. Pediatrics 42: 492
Auricchio S, Rubino A, Murset G 1965 Intestinal glycosidase activities in the human embryo, fetus and newborn. Pediatrics 35: 944–964
Barr R G, Levine M D, Watkins J B 1979 Recurrent abdominal pain in childhood due to lactose intolerance. New England Journal of Medicine 300: 1449–1452
Bayless T M, Paige D M 1979 Lactose intolerance. Current Concepts in Nutrition 8: 79–90
Bayless T M, Rosensweig N S 1966 A racial difference in incidence of lactase deficiency. Journal of the American Medical Association 197: 968–972
Bedine M S, Bayless T M 1973 Intolerance of small amounts of lactose by individuals with low lactase levels. Gastroenterology 65: 735–743
Boellner S W, Beard A G, Panos T 1965 Impairment of intestinal hydrolysis of lactose in newborn infants. Pediatrics 36: 542–550
Bolin T D, Davis A E, Seah C S, Chua K L, Yong M B V, Kho K M, Siak C L, Jacob E 1970 Lactose intolerance in Singapore. Gastroenterology 59: 76–84
Bond J H, Levitt M D 1976a Quantitative measurement of lactose absorption. Gastroenterology 70: 1058–1062
Bond J H, Levitt M D 1976b Fate of soluble carbohydrate in the colon of rat and man. Journal of Clinical Investigation 57: 1156–64
Book L S, Herbst J J, Jung A L 1976 Carbohydrate malabsorption in necrotising enterocolitis. Pediatrics 57: 201–204
Bowie M D 1975 Effect of lactose-induced diarrhoea on absorption of nitrogen and fat. Archives of Disease in Childhood 50: 363–366
Bowie M D, Barbezat G O, Hansen J D L 1967 Carbohydrate absorption in malnourished children. American Journal of Clinical Nutrition 20: 89–97
Bowie M D, Brinkman G L, Hansen J D L 1965 Acquired disaccharide intolerance in malnutrition. Journal of Pediatrics 66: 1083–1091

Brand J C, Gracey M, Spargo R, Dutton S 1983 Lactose malabsorption in Australian Aborigines. American Journal of Clinical Nutrition 37: 449–52

Brand J, Mitchell J D 1980 Faecal fat losses and cow's milk lactose. Lancet i: 207

Brown K H 1981 Milk supplement for children in the tropics. In: Paige D M, Bayless T M (eds) Lactose digestion: clinical and nutritional implications The Johns Hopkins University Press, Baltimore & London

Bullen C L, Tearle P V, Stewart M G 1977 The effect of 'humanised' milks and supplemented breast feeding on the faecal flora of infants. Journal of Medical Microbiology 10: 403–13

Calloway D H, Murphy E L, Baver D 1969 Determination of lactose intolerance by breath analysis. American Journal of Digestive Disease 14: 811–815

Chalfin D, Holt P H 1967 Lactase deficiency in ulcerative colitis, regional enteritis and viral hepatitis. American Journal of Digestive Diseases 12: 81–87

Chandra R K, Pawa R R, Ghai O P 1968 Sugar intolerance in malnourished infants and children. British Medical Journal 4: 611–613

Christopher M, Bayless T M 1971 The role of the small bowel and colon in lactose-induced diarrhea. Gastroenterology 60: 805–52

Cook G C (undated manuscript) Incidence and clinical features of specific hypolactasia in Adult man. Reprint from Symposia of the Swedish Nutrition Foundation XI

Cook G C 1967 Lactase activity in newborn and infant Baganda. British Medical Journal 1: 527–530

Cook G C, Asp N G, Dahlqvist A 1973 Activities of brush border lactase, acid β-galactosidase and hetero-β-galactosidase in the jejunum of the Zambian African. Gastroenterology 64: 405–410

Cook G C, Dahlqvist A 1968 Jejunal hetero-β-galactosidase activities in Ugandans with lactase deficiency. Gastroenterology 55: 328–332

Cook G C, Kajubi S K 1966 Tribal incidence of lactase deficiency in Uganda. Lancet i: 725–730

Dagan R, Gorodischer R, Moses S, Margolis C 1980 Lactose-free formula for infantile diarrhoea. Lancet i: 207

Dahlqvist A 1964 Method for the assay of intestinal disaccharidases. Analytical Biochemistry 7: 18–25

Dahlqvist A 1977 The basic aspects of the chemical background of lactase deficiency. In: Barltrop D (ed) Paediatric implications for some adult disorders. Report of the fourth Unigate Paediatric Worshop, Fellowship of Postgraduate Medicine, London, p 57–62

Davidson A G F, Mullinger M 1970 Reducing substances in neonatal stools detected by Clinitest. Pediatrics 46: 632–635

Debongnie J C, Newcomer A D, McGill D B, Phillips S F 1979 Absorption of nutrients in lactase deficiency. Digestive Diseases and Sciences 24: 225–231

Doell R G, Kretchmer N 1962 Studies of small intestine during development: 1. Distribution and activity of β-galactosidase. Biochimica et Biophysica Acta 62: 353–362

Dubois R S, Roy C C, Fulginiti V A, Merrill D A, Murray R L 1970 Disaccharidase deficiency in children with immunologic deficits. Journal of Pediatrics 76: 377–385

Dunphy J V, Littman A, Hammond J B, Forstner G, Dahlqvist A, Crane R K 1965 Intestinal lactase deficits in adults. Gastroenterology 49: 12–21

Gall D G 1980 Viral gastroenteritis. In: Lifshitz F (ed) Clinical disorders in clinical gastroenterology and nutrition, New York, Marcel Dekker, p 293–99

Garza C, Scrimshaw N S 1976 Relationship of lactose tolerance to milk intolerance in young children. American Journal of Clinical Nutrition 29: 192–196

Gilat T, Russo S, Gelman-Malachi E, Aldon T A M 1972 Lactase in man: A non-adaptable enzyme. Gastroenterology 62: 1125–27

Gray G M, Walter W H J, Colver E H 1968 Persistent deficiency of intestinal lactase in apparently cured tropical sprue. Gastroenterology 54: 552–558

Gudmand-Hoyer E, Jarnum S 1969 Lactose malabsorption in Greenland Eskimos. Acta Medica Scandinavica 186: 235–237

Gyorgy P 1953 A hitherto unrecognized biochemical difference between human milk and cow's milk. Pediatrics 11: 98–108

Holmes I H, Schangl R D, Rodger S, Ruck B J, Gust I D, Bishop R F, Barnes G L 1976 Is lactase the receptor and uncoating enzyme for infantile enteritis (rota) viruses? Lancet i: 1387–88

Holzel A, Schwarz V, Sutcliffe K W 1959 Defective lactose absorption causing malnutrition in infancy. Lancet 1126–1128

Hoskova A, Sabacky J, Mrskos A, Pospisil R 1980 Severe lactose intolerance with lactosuria and vomiting. Archives of Disease in Childhood 55: 304–316

Hyams J S, Krause P J, Gleason P A 1981 Lactose malabsorption following rotavirus infection in young children. The Journal of Pediatrics 99: 916–918

Jarrett E C, Holman G H 1966 Lactose absorption in the premature infant. Archives of Disease in Childhood 41: 525–527

Jersky J, Kinsley R H 1967 Lactase deficiency in the South African Bantu. South African Medical Journal 41: 1194–1196

Johnson J D, Kretchmer N, Simoons F J 1974 Lactose malabsorption: its biology and history. Advances in Pediatrics 21: 197–237

Johnson J D, Simoons F J, Hurwitz R, Grange A, Mitchell C H, Sinatra F R et al 1977 Lactose malabsorption among the Pima Indians of Arizona. Gastroenterology 73: 1299–1304

Johnson J D, Simoons P J, Hurwitz R, Grange A, Sinatra F R, Sunshine P et al 1978 Lactose malabsorption among adult Indians of the Great Basin and American Southwest. American Journal of Clinical Nutrition 31: 381–87

Johnson J L, McBee R J 1967 The porcupine cecal fermentation. Journal of Nutrition 91: 540–46

Jussila J 1969 Milk intolerance and lactose malabsorption in hospital patients and young servicemen in Finland. Annals of Clinical Research 1: 199

Kapikian A Z, Kim H W, Wyatt R E, Cline W L, Arrobio J O, Brandt C D, et al 1976 Human reovirus-like agent as the major pathogen associated with 'winter' gastroenteritis in hospitalized infants and young children. New England Journal of Medicine 294: 965–72

Kerry K R, Anderson C M 1964 A ward test for sugar in faeces. Lancet ii: 981–982

Keusch G T, Troncale F J, Miller L H, Promadhat V, Anderson P R, 1965 Acquired lactose malabsorption in Thai children. Pediatrics 43: 540–45

Keusch G T, Troncale F J, Thararamara B, Prinyamont P, Anderson P R, Bhamarapravath 1969 Lactase deficiency in Thailand: Effect of prolonged lactase feeding. American Journal of Clinical Nutrition 22: 638–641

King F 1972 Intolerance to lactose in mothers' milk? Lancet ii: 335

Kretchmer N 1977 The geography and biology of lactose digestion and malabsorption. In: Barltrop D (ed) Paediatric implication of some adult disorders. Report of the Fourth Unigate Paediatric Workshop, Fellowship of Postgraduate Medicine, London, p 65–70

Kretchmer N, Ransome-Kuti O, Hurwitz R, Dungy C, Alakija W 1971 Intestinal absorption of lactose in Nigerian ethnic groups. Lancet ii: 392–395

Kretchmer N, Sunshine P 1967 Intestinal disaccharidase deficiency in the sea lion. Gastroenterology 53: 123–129

Launiala K 1968 The mechanism of diarrhoea in congenital disaccharide malabsorption. Acta Paediatrica Scandinavica 57: 425–432

Leichter J, Tolensky A F 1975 Effect of dietary lactose on the absorption of protein, fat and calcium in the post weaning rat. American Journal of Clinical Nutrition 28: 238–241

Levin B, Abraham J M, Burgess E A, Wallis P G 1970 Congenital lactose malabsorption. Archives of Disease in Childhood 45: 175–177

Liebman W M 1979 Recurrent abdominal pain in children: lactose and sucrose intolerance. A prospective study. Pediatrics 64: 43–45

Lifshitz F 1966 Congenital lactase deficiency. Journal of Pediatrics 69: 229–37

Lifshitz F, Wapnir R A, Wehman H J, Hawkins R L, Diaz-Bensussen S 1974 Enteric microflora effects on intestinal transport of carbohydrates. Federation Proceedings 33: 673

Lisker R, Aguilar L, Lares I, Cravioto J 1980 Double-blind study of milk lactose intolerance in a group of rural and urban children. American Journal of Clinical Nutrition 3: 1049–1053

Lubos M C, Gerrard J W, Buchan D J 1967 Disaccharidase activities in milk sensitive and celiac patients. Pediatrics 70: 325–333

McGill D B, Newcomer A D 1967 Comparison of venous and capillary blood samples in lactose tolerance testing. Gastroenterology 53: 371–374

Maclean J R W C, Fink B 1981 Lactose digestion by premature infants: Hydrogen breath test results versus estimates of energy loss. In: Paige D M, Bayless T M (eds) Lactose digestion: clinical and nutritional implications. The Johns Hopkins University Press, Baltimore & London

McMichael H B, Webb J, Dawson A M 1965 Lactase deficiency in adults: Cause of functional diarrhoea. Lancet i: 717–720

Mitchell K J, Bayless T M, Paige D M, Goodgame R W, Huang S S 1975 Intolerance of eight ounces of milk in healthy lactose-intolerance teenagers. Paediatrics 56: 716–721

Neale G 1968 The diagnosis, incidence and significance of disaccharidase deficiency in adults. Proceedings of the Royal Society of Medicine 61: 109

Nose O, Iida Y, Kai H, Harada T, Ogawa I, Yabunchi H 1979 Breath hydrogen test for detecting lactose malabsorption in infants and children: Prevalence of lactose malabsorption in Japanese children and adults. Archives of Disease in Childhood 54: 436–4440

Olatunbosun D A, Adadevoh B K 1972 Lactose intolerance in Nigerian children. Acta Paediatrica Scandinavica 61: 715–719

Paige D M 1981 Lactose malabsorption in children: In: Paige D M, Bayless T M (eds) Lactose digestion: clinical and nutritional implications. The Johns Hopkins University Press, Baltimore & London

Paige D M, Bayless T H, Huang S S, Wexler R 1975 Lactose hydrolysed milk. American Journal of Clinical Nutrition 28: 818–822

Phillips S F 1981 Lactose malabsorption and gastrointestinal function. Effects of gastrointestinal transit and the absorption of other nutrients. In: Paige D M, Bayless T M (eds) Lactose digestion: clinical and nutritional implications. The Johns Hopkins University Press, Baltimore & London

Pirk F, Skala I 1972 Functional response of the digestive tract to the ingestion of milk in subjects suffering from lactose intolerance. Digestion 5: 89–99

Plimmer R H A 1906 On the presence of lactase in the intestine of animals and on the adaptation of the intestine to lactose. Journal of Physiology 35: 20–31

Prinsloo J G, Wittmann W, Pretorious P J, Kruger A, Fellingham S A 1969 Effect of different sugars on diarrhoea of acute kwashiorkor. Archives of Disease in Childhood 44: 593–599

Ransome-Kuti O, Kretchmer N, Johnson J D et al 1975 A genetic study of lactose digestion in Nigerian families. Gastroenterology 68: 431–436

Ruppin H, Bar-Meir S, Soergel K H, Wood C M, Steff J J 1980 Absorption of short-chain fatty acids by the colon. Gastroenterology 76: 1500–1507

Sabre M, Kabrashi K 1979 Lactose tolerance in Iran. American Journal of Clinical Nutrition 32: 1948–1954

Savilahti E, Launiala K, Kuitunen P 1983 Congenital lactase deficiency. Archives of Disease in Childhood 58: 246–252

Simoons F J 1973 New light on ethnic differences in adult lactose intolerance. Digestive Disorders 18: 595–611

Sterk V V, Kretchmer N 1964 Studies of small intestine during development. IV. Digestion of lactose as related to lactosuria in the rabbit. Pediatrics 34: 609

Strickland A, Garza C, Nichols B 1979 Formula effects on growth after diarrhea. American Journal of Clinical Nutrition 32: 937

Sunshine P, Kretchmer N 1964 Studies of small intestine during development. III. Infantile diarrhea associated with intolerance to disaccharides. Pediatrics 34: 38–50

Tandon R, Mandell H, Spiro H M, Thayer W R 1971 Lactose intolerance in Jewish patients with ulcerative colitis. Digestive Diseases 16: 845–848

Tejani N, Lifshitz F, Harper R G 1979 The response to an oral glucose load during convalescent from hypoxia in newborn infants. The Journal of Pediatrics 94: 792–96

Torres-Pinedo R, Lavastida M, Rivera C L, Rodriguez H, Ortiz A 1966 Studies in infants diarrhea: I.A. Comparison of the effects of milk feeding and intravenous therapy on the composition and volume of the stool and urine. Journal of Clinical Investigation 45: 469–480

Watkins J B 1981 Recurrent abdominal pain: Role of lactose intolerance: In: Paige D M, Bayless T M (eds) Lactose digestion: clinical and nutritional implications. The Johns Hopkins University Press, Baltimore & London, p 173–181

Welsh J D 1970 Isolated lactase deficiency in humans: Report on 100 patients. Medicine 49: 257–277

Welsh J D, Hall W H 1977 Gastric emptying of lactose and milk in subjects with lactose malabsorption. American Journal of Digestive Diseases 22: 1060–63

Welsh J D, Rohrer G V, Walker A 1966 Human intestinal lactase intestinal activity. 1. Normal individuals. Archives of Internal Medicine 117: 488–494

Weser E, Ruben W, Ross L, Sleisenger M H 1965 Lactase deficiency in patients with the irritable colon syndrome. New England Journal of Medicine 273: 1070

Wharton B, Howells G, Phillips I 1968 Diarrhoea in kwashiorkor. British Medical Journal 2: 608–613

Young M G, Manoharan K, Mickelson O 1970 Nutritional contribution of volatile fatty acids from the caecum of rats. Journal of Nutrition 100: 545–550

Zeigler E E, Fomon S J 1980 Lactose and mineral absorption in infancy. Pediatric Research 14: 513

Infant feeding practices

There are two main ways in which feeding practices may modify diarrhoeal morbidity and growth patterns during infancy, both of considerable topical interest and both associated with some degree of controversy. In this chapter an attempt will be made to identify acceptable generalizations and to indicate those areas where there appear to be conflicting data or where there are important inadequacies in our basic knowledge.

BREAST OR BOTTLE?

The first and most obvious issue is whether infants are fed from birth on human breast milk or on some form of cows' milk substitute. This has important implications in terms of morbidity and also of growth. There is a wealth of literature comparing the morbidity of bottle-fed children with that of breast-fed and in the underpriviledged third world situation a consistent pattern is observed in which bottle-fed children suffer significantly more frequent gastrointestinal infections (Grantham-McGregor & Back 1970, Plank &Milanesi 1973). In addition, some workers have shown a similar pattern of increased rates of extra-intestinal infection, usually upper respiratory infections, as in one series (Chandra 1979) which covered both a developing country (rural India) and an industralized one (urban Canada). On the same theme Cunningham (1981) reviewed a number of studies carried out in the West during this century and concluded that breast-feeding reduced morbidity and mortality from respiratory as well as diarrhoeal diseases, particularly in the period prior to World War II, and mostly in the younger infant age group. The same trend with respect to severe infections had been noted by Wray (1978) at least up until recent years. These findings were also supported by the study of Larsen & Homer (1978) who found a significant preponderance of young bottle-fed infants hospitalized for severe gastroenteritis in their middle-class Californian population.

The concept that breast-fed children enjoy lower morbidity rates than bottle-fed in the relatively priviledged environment of the industralized countries has however been challenged by Sauls (1979). He highlighted the failure of studies to make adequate allowance for the almost inevitable pres-

119

ence of many confounding variables, the most obvious of which include education and literacy, social class and the home environment. Because of these problems he felt that one could not make definitive conclusions from currently available data as to whether breast-feeding significantly reduced morbidity in industrialized societies.

Though this may be an overstatement it is a timely reminder that in situations where people enjoy an increasingly high standard of living and education the differences in morbidity may be becoming less marked and attention to such details becomes correspondingly more important. For example, one recent study of a large series of children in the United Kingdom failed to show significant differences in the rates of severe morbidity in breast- and bottle-fed children in the first year of life (Taylor et al 1982), after controlling for a large number of variables. Even then, however, there was a trend towards higher rates of gastrointestinal infection amongst bottle-fed children. Perhaps the best insight into the current situation in the industrialized countries is afforded by the work of Fergusson et al (1981) in New Zealand who concluded that protection by breast-feeding against gastroenteritis was detectable only during the first four months of life. The same authors were unable to demonstrate any difference with respect to respiratory infections when taking into account the other variables studied.

This relatively minor area of ambiguity is perhaps unsurprising when one considers that in many developed countries the incidence and duration of breast-feeding tends to be positively correlated with higher levels of maternal education and higher social class as documented in the UK (Martin 1978) and in Australia (Boulton & Coote 1979). This group of mothers might reasonably be expected to be successful in avoiding many of the more obvious problems associated with bottle-feeding, such as contamination and incorrect mixing referred to latter.

The picture is very different in the developing countries of the world where it is the urban middle- and upper-income groups who abandon the breast in favour of bottle-feeding (World Health Organization 1981a) in a home environment which may still present significant hazards to their infants. Fortunately this trend is not as widespread and prevalent in the third world as one might sometimes imagine and, following an extensive overview of international feeding practices, Thomson & Black (1975) concluded that breast-feeding was most common and longest sustained in the most economically disadvantaged and 'traditional' communities.

The relative freedom from gastrointestinal infection of breast-fed children can probably be explained largely by two main mechanisms. One is negative, namely the relatively low exposure to and consumption of gut pathogens of the exclusively breast-fed child. The second is the positive protection afforded by the various antimicrobial mechanisms which have been demonstrated in breast milk. Our understanding of these is still imperfect and it is not always possible to determine which aspect is more important even where quite specific studies have been carried out, such as that in Bahrain on cholera during infancy (Gunn et al 1979).

The subject of host defence mechanisms in breast milk is a major one in its own right and the reader is referred elsewhere for details of this nature. Fresh human milk has been used both in prevention (Narayanan et al 1980) and treatment of gastrointestinal infection in the neonatal period. The degree of protection in natural circumstances is however variable depending on the individual mother, the stage of lactation (i.e. the age of the infant) and the extent to which other fluids or foods are consumed by the infant. In a specific study in which levels of antibacterial activity of mothers' milk directed in vitro against *Escherichia coli* were related to the in vivo diarrhoeal experience of the recipient infant, Rowland et al (1980) concluded that in a minority of cases protection appeared to be virtually complete for the first half of infancy. If correct this probably represents the upper end of the age range. In a broad review already mentioned above (Thomson & Black 1975) the authors concluded that prolonged breast-feeding was unlikely to prevent infections among older infants in heavily contaminated third world environments. Though anti-infective factors present in breast milk may prevent symptoms in early infancy they may not prevent carriage and excretion of potential gut pathogens following exposure, nor indeed the negative inpact of these organisms on growth (Mata et al 1972).

WEANING

One constraint on the completeness of protection by breast-feeding may be the age at which weaning is initiated. Plank & Milanesi (1973) found no difference in the morbidity experienced by bottle-fed and partially breast-fed infants.

Before proceeding further it is necessary to clarify the terminology as the use of the word 'weaning' is open to differing interpretations depending on the circumstances in which it is applied. Thus, in the infant raised from birth on cows' milk substitute, weaning may correctly have been said to have occurred at birth. Others apply the term to the time when solids or semi-solids are added to the diet of the cows' milk-fed infant but this has little to recommend it from a physiological point of view. In this description *weaning* refers to the introduction and regular consumption of additional foods by an otherwise breast-fed infant. The *weaning period* starts with the use of such feeds and ceases when breast-feeding is finally terminated. The use of drinks of 'raw' water in the otherwise breast-fed child is ignored in this context. Though there is no physiological justification for this widespread practice (Armelini & Gonzalez 1979), it appears unlikely that it would normally contribute a large infective bolus to the gastrointestinal tract of the breast-fed infant nor substantially interfere with the process of suckling and lactation.

The weaning period has long been recognized as one of high risk (Welbourn 1955, Gordon et al 1963). The nature and timing of the weaning process is likely to have a bearing both on nutritional intake and on the amount of gastrointestinal infection experienced during infancy; both of these factors may independently exert a profound effect on growth in a variety of ways. Hence the whole question of weaning strategy is of fundamental importance when considering the problem of malnutrition and diarrhoeal illness in the third world. Rowland et al (1978) coined the phrase 'the weanling's dilemma' attempting to focus attention on various aspects of this problem which are presented in simplified form in Figure 8.1. This scenario has been further examined by Waterlow (1981).

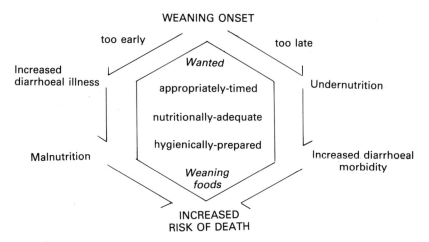

Fig. 8.1 The weanling's dilemma

Logically the timing of the introduction of additional foods to the diet of the breast-fed child should be determined by the quantity and quality and duration of production of the mother's milk and the adequacy of the infant's growth in relation to this. It seems reasonably clear that there is a positive relationship between maternal nutritional status and weight gain during pregnancy, particularly the last trimester, and the outcome of pregnancy i.e. birthweight (Habicht et al 1975). These variables also appear to be related to lactation performance, including the quantity, quality and duration of production of breast-milk (Whitehead et al 1978, Wray 1978, Mardones-Santander 1979, Prentice 1980).

Armed with various data on infant size, growth velocity, breast-milk intake volumes and nutritional content, various authors have attempted to arrive at a figure for the age at which exclusive breast-feeding can no longer adequately sustain growth. In practice this sort of approach is bedevilled at every point by a number of quite fundamental areas of ignorance such as the lack of appropriate reference growth standards in early infancy (Rowland et al 1981, Whitehead & Paul 1984), a recent reappraisal of energy requirements in infancy (Whitehead et al 1981), the inherent inaccuracy stemming from assigning a fixed value for the energy content of milk from different mothers (Prentice et al 1981) and the relatively recent development of technology permitting the accurate assessment in the home or field of breast-milk intakes over prolonged periods of time (Coward et al 1979, Coward et al 1982). It is hardly surprising therefore that final estimates for the nutritional adequacy of exclusive breast-feeding have ranged from as low as two months (Waterlow & Thomson 1979) to as high as six months (Jelliffe & Jelliffe 1979). In practice we recognise the fallacy of trying to make generalizations in a situation where the assessment should ideally be made on the basis of monitoring each individual's progress (Scrimshaw & Underwood 1980, Whitehead & Paul 1981). Taking a very different approach in a study of urban Gambian children, it was found (Rowland et al 1984) that infants who were started on weaning prior to three months of age showed no particular pattern of preceding size or growth in weight and in these children weaning onset tended to be followed by growth faltering. Where mothers introduced weaning foods later than three months they tended to start with the smaller, slower-growing infants who showed no resultant growth impairment.

In this particular study, moreover, there was no evidence to support the fear that the early initiation of weaning necessarily leads to premature cessation of breast-feeding. In fact, though this belief is commonplace, it is clear that breast-feeding may be systematically supplemented even within the first three months of life, sometimes with bottled feeds, yet be successfully maintained for a year or more later (Viseshakul et al 1977, Kardjati et al 1978, Whitehead et al 1978, Van Steenbergen et al 1981, Gussler & Mock 1983). It must be said, however, that the implication of weaning onset in terms of quantity of breast milk consumed as opposed to duration of lactation is not yet clear; at least one study in the United Kingdom has shown clear evidence of quite profound changes in maternal hormonal profile following abruptly on the introduction of supplementary foods to the infant (Howie et al 1981) and these may affect milk production.

In the third world any foodstuff other than breast-milk fed to infants, either as a replacement or a supplement, commercial or traditional, bottle or spoon-fed, is likely to be nutritionally inadequate (Hudson et al 1980, Van Steenbergen et al 1981) and bacteriologically contaminated (Surjono et al 1980, Barrell & Rowland 1980). Though a number of studies have failed to demonstrate a general relationship between weaning food contamination and level of diarrhoeal morbidity (Surjono et al 1980, Lloyd-Evans et al 1984) few people could doubt that this was an important epidemiological factor. The specific hazards associated with the supplanting of breast-feeding by bottle-fed commercial products have been examined in detail (Brown 1973, Jelliffe 1979). In recent years there has been a major reappraisal of the activities of the infant food industry (ICIFI 1978) and considerable steps have been taken to regulate the use of such products both in developing and industrialized countries (WHO 1981b).

CONCLUSION

How successful is the outcome of current breast-feeding promotion? There are many examples of a resurgence of breast-feeding at least in the industrialized countries such as the United States of America (Martinez & Nalezienski 1981), the United Kingdom (Martin & Monk 1982), and Australia (Lawson et al 1978). The potential benefits of supplementing the diet of selected pregnant mothers have been demonstrated (Kielmann et al 1978, Prentice et al 1983) but the further knowledge and understanding necessary for the widespread application of this is yet to be achieved (Habicht & Yarbrough 1980). The problems of safely and effectively complementing the diet of the breast-fed third world infant remain largely unsolved (Scrimshaw &Underwood 1980). The problem of the low energy density and viscosity of traditional weaning foods (Ljungqvist et al 1981) has long been recognized and one must welcome and applaud the few initiatives that are being shown (Brandtzaeg et al 1981) to develop village technology to improve these aspects leading to improved bioavailability, and quite possibly hygienic qualities, of local supplementary weaning foods. Only when these general strategies have been further refined and applied in conjunction with improved immunoprophylactic measures against specific diarrhoeal agents may one expect to see major reductions in diarrhoeal morbidity and malnutrition in the environment inhabited by so many third world children today.

The reader's attention is directed to an excellent annotated bibliography on infant and young child feeding recently compiled by Ashworth et al (1982). This is selective and gives precedence to the more recent publications on the subject and covers many of the issues raised in this book.

REFERENCES

Armelini P A, Gonzalez C F 1979 Breast feeding and fluid intake in a hot climate. Clinical Pediatrics 18: 424–425

Ashworth A, Allen S R, Fookes G A 1982 Infant and child feeding — a selected annotated bibliography. Early Human Development (Supplement) 6: 1–168

Barrell R A E, Rowland M G M 1980 Commercial milk products and indigenous weaning foods in a rural West African environment — a bacteriological perspective. Journal of Hygiene, Cambridge 84: 191–202

Boulton T J C, Coote L M 1979 Nutritional studies during early childhood. II Feeding practices during infancy, and their relationship to socio-economic and cultural factors. Australian Paediatric Journal 15: 81–86

Brandtzaeg B, Malleshi N G, Svanberg U, Desikachar H S B, Mellander O 1981 Dietary bulk as a limiting factor for nutrient intake — with special reference to the feeding of pre-school children. III Studies of malted flour from ragi, sorghum and green gram. Journal of Tropical Pediatrics 27: 184–189

Brown R E 1973 Breastfeeding in modern times. American Journal of Clinical Nutrition 26: 556–562

Chandra R K 1979 Prospective studies of the effect of breastfeeding on incidence of infection and allergy. Acta Paediatrica Scandinavica 68: 691–694

Coward W A, Cole T J, Sawyer M B, Prentice A M 1982 Breast-milk intake measurement in mixed-fed infants by administration of deuterium oxide to their mothers. Human Nutrition: Clinical Nutrition 36C: 141–148

Coward W A, Whitehead R G, Sawyer M B, Prentice A M, Evans J 1979 New method for measuring milk intakes in breast-fed babies. Lancet ii: 13–14

Cunningham A S 1981 Breastfeeding and morbidity in industralized countries: an update. In: Jelliffe D B, Jelliffe E F P (eds) Advances in international maternal and child health, vol 1. Oxford Medical Publications, Oxford, p 128–168

Fergusson D M, Horwood L J, Shannon F T, Taylor B 1981 Breast-feeding, gastrointestinal and lower respiratory illness in the first two years. Australian Paediatric Journal 17: 191–195

Gordon J E, Chitkara I D, Wyon J B 1963 Weanling diarrhea. American Journal of Medical Science 245: 345–377

Grantham-McGregor S M, Back E H 1970 Breastfeeding in Kingston, Jamaica. Archives of Disease in Childhood 45: 404–409

Gunn R A, Kimball A M, Pollard R A, Feely J C, Feldman R A, Dutta S R, Matthew P P, Mahmood R A, Levine M M 1979 Bottle feeding as a risk factor for cholera in infants. Lancet ii: 730–732

Gussler J D, Mock N 1983 A comparative description of infant feeding practices in Zaire, The Philippines and St Kitts-Nevis. Ecology of Food and Nutrition 13: 75–85

Habicht J-P, Delgado H, Yarbrough C, Klein R E 1975 Repercussions of lactation on nutritional status of mother and infant. In: Proceedings of the IXth International Congress of Nutrition, Mexico 1972, vol 2. S Karger, Basel, p 106–114

Habicht J-P, Yarbrough C 1980 Efficiency in selecting pregnant women for food supplementation during pregnancy. In: Aebi H, Whitehead R G (eds) Maternal nutrition during pregnancy and lactation. Hans Huber Publishers, Bern, p 314–336

Howie P W, McNeilly A S, Houston M J, Cook A, Boyle H 1981 Effect of supplementary food on suckling patterns and ovarian activity during lactation. British Medical Journal 283: 757–759

Hudson G J, John P M W, Paul A A 1980 Variation in the composition of Gambian foods: The importance of water in relation to energy and protein content. Ecology of Food and Nutrition 10: 9–17

ICIFI 1978 International Council of Infant Food Industries. Its aims and progress. Lancet i: 1250–1252

Jelliffe D B, Jelliffe E F P 1979 Adequacy of breastfeeding. Lancet ii: 691–692

Jelliffe E F P 1979 The impact of the food industry on the nutritional status of young children in developing countries. In: Mayer J, Dwyer J T (eds) Food and nutrition policy in a changing world. Oxford University Press, New York, p 197–222

Kardjati S, Kusin J A, De With C, Sudigbia I K 1978 Feeding practices, nutritional status and mortality in pre-school children in rural East Java, Indonesia. Tropical Geographical Medicine 30: 359–371

Kielmann A A, Taylor C E, Parker R L 1978 The Narangwal Nutrition Study: a summary review, American Journal of Clinical Nutrition 31: 2040–2052

Larsen S A, Homer D R 1978 Relation of breast- versus bottle-feeding to hospitalization for gastroenteritis in a middle-class US population. Journal of Pediatrics 92: 417–418

Lawson J S, Mays C A, Oliver T I 1978 The return to breast-feeding. Medical Journal of Australia 2: 229–230

Ljungqvist B G, Mellander O, Svanberg U S O 1981 Dietary bulk as a limiting factor for nutrient intake in pre-school children. I A problem description. Journal of Tropical Pediatrics 27: 68–73

Lloyd-Evans N, Pickering H A, Goh S G J, Rowland M G M 1984 Food and water hygiene and diarrhoea in young Gambian children: a limited case control study. Transactions of the Royal Society of Tropical Medicine and Hygiene 78: 209–211

Mardones-Santander F 1979 History of breastfeeding in Chile. United Nations University Food and Nutrition Bulletin 1: 15–22

Martin J 1978 Infant feeding 1975: attitudes and practice in England and Wales. Her Majesty's Stationery Office, London

Martin J, Monk J 1982 Infant feeding 1980. Office of Population Censuses and Surveys, London

Martinez G A, Nalezienski J P 1981 1980 Up-date: recent trend in breastfeeding. Pediatrics 67: 260–263

Mata L J, Urrutia J J, Abertazzi C, Pellecer O, Arellano E 1972 Influence of recurrent infections on nutrition and growth of children in Guatemala. American Journal of Clinical Nutrition 25: 1267–1275

Narayanan I, Prakash K, Bala S, Verma R K, Gujral V V 1980 Partial supplementation with expressed breast-milk for prevention of infection in low birth-weight infants. Lancet ii: 561–562

Plank S J, Milanesi M L 1973 Infant feeding and infant mortality in rural Chile. Bulletin of the World Health Organization 48: 203–210

Prentice A, Prentice A M, Whitehead R G 1981 Breast-milk fat concentrations of rural African women 2. Long-term variations within a community. British Journal of Nutrition 45: 495–503

Prentice A M 1980 Variations in maternal dietary intake, birthweight and breast-milk output in The Gambia. In: Aebi H, Whitehead R G (eds) Maternal nutrition during pregnancy and lactation. Hans Huber Publishers, Bern, p 167–183

Prentice A M, Whitehead R G, Watkinson M, Lamb W H, Cole T J 1983 Prenatal dietary supplementation of African women and birth-weight. Lancet i: 489–492

Rowland M G M, Barrell R A E, Whitehead R G 1978 Bacterial contamination in traditional Gambian weaning foods. Lancet i: 136–138

Rowland M G M, Cole T J, Tully M, Dolby J M, Honour P 1980 Bacteriostasis of Escherichia coli by milk. VI. The in-vitro bacteriostatic property of Gambian mothers' breast milk in relation to the in-vivo protection of their infants against diarrhoeal disease. Journal of Hygiene, Cambridge 85: 405–413

Rowland M G M, Goh S G J, Tulloch S, Dunn D T, Hayes R J 1984 Growth and weaning in urban Gambian infants. In: Eekels R, Ransome-Kuti O (eds) Child Health in the Tropics. Sixth Nutricia Symposium. Martinus Nijhof Publishers, The Hauge, in press

Rowland M G M, Paul A A, Whitehead R G 1981 Lactation and infant nutrition. British Medical Bulletin 37: 77–82

Sauls H S 1979 Potential effect of demographic and other variables in studies comparing morbidity of breast-fed and bottle-fed infants. Pediatrics 64: 523–527

Scrimshaw N S, Underwood B 1980 Timely and appropriate complementary feeding of the breast-fed infant — an overview. United Nations University Food and Nutrition Bulletin 2: 19–22

Surjono D, Ismadi S D, Surwadji, Rohde J E 1980 Bacterial contamination and dilution of milk in infant feeding bottles. Journal of Tropical Paediatrics 26: 58–61

Taylor B, Wadsworth J, Golding J, Butler N 1982 Breastfeeding, bronchitis and admissions for lower-respiratory illness and gastroenteritis during the first five years. Lancet i: 1227–1229

Thomson A M, Black A E 1975 Nutritional aspects of human lactation. Bulletin of the World Health Organization 52: 163–177

Van Steenbergen W M, Kusin J A, Van Rens M M 1981 Lactation performance of Akamba mothers, Kenya. Breastfeeding behaviour, breast milk yield and composition. Journal of Tropical Pediatrics 27: 155–161

Viseshakul D, Techakaisaya D, Chularojmoutri V, Premwatana P, Rajatasilpin A 1977 Growth rate, feeding practices, dietary intake of Thai infants under three years old and of two Bangkok slum areas. Journal of the Medical Association of Thailand 60: 551–558

Waterlow J C 1981 Observations on the suckling's dilemma — a personal view. Journal of Human Nutrition 35: 85–98

Waterlow J C, Thomson A M 1979 Observations on the adequacy of breastfeeding. Lancet ii: 238–242

Welbourn H F 1955 The danger period during weaning. Parts I, II, III. Journal of Tropical Paediatrics 1: 34–46, 98–111, 161–173

Whitehead R G, Paul A A 1981 Infant growth and human milk requirements. A fresh approach. Lancet ii: 161–163

Whitehead R G, Paul A A 1984 Growth charts and the assessment of infant feeding practices in the western world and in developing countries. Early Human Development 8: in press

Whitehead R G, Rowland M G M, Hutton M, Prentice A M, Müller E, Paul A 1978 Factors influencing lactation performance in rural Gambian mothers. Lancet ii: 178–181

World Health Organization 1981a Contempor-ary patterns of breast-feeding. Report of the WHO Collaborative Study on breast-feeding. World Health Organization, Geneva, p 211

World Health Organization 1981b International Code of marketing of breast-milk substitutes. World Health Organization, Geneva, p 36

Wray J D 1978 Maternal nutrition, breastfeeding and infant survival. In: Mosley W H (ed) Nutrition and human reproduction. Plenum, New York, p 197–229

Prospects for antidiarrhoeal therapy in acute diarrhoeas

INTRODUCTION

Over the past decade oral rehydration therapy has become accepted as the treatment of choice for acute diarrhoea in the developing countries. This has been a major advance in the effort to reduce mortality associated with diarrhoea. However, in cases of severe purging, oral therapy may not be adequate to maintain hydration, and, in addition, intravenous therapy may not be practical, or even possible in many areas. Therefore, the need for a safe, effective antidiarrhoeal agent is clear.

A long list of compounds has evolved from the search for the ideal antidiarrhoeal drug. Such a drug should have a high degree of activity, be effective orally, target its action on the intestine without systemic absorption or systemic effect, have no effect on a normally functioning gut and have a mechanism of action which is well understood. In this chapter we will review the current knowledge regarding the mechanisms of action and effectiveness of currently available antidiarrhoeal agents and will consider the potential of various experimental compounds. As the title of this chapter suggests, no specific antidiarrhoeal agent can be recommended at this time for routine therapy in the acute diarrhoeas. Instead we offer possibilities; antidiarrhoeal agents which may be useful as adjuncts to rehydration therapy.

ANTIMICROBIAL AGENTS

Antimicrobial agents are not considered to be antidiarrhoeal drugs. However, since a significant proportion of acute diarrhoeas are the result of bacterial infections (Black et al 1980, Black et al 1982), it would seem logical that antimicrobial agents directed at eliminating the pathogenic organisms would be the most effective means of controlling diarrhoea. In theory this is only true if the specific pathogen and its antibiotic sensitivity are known and if treatment significantly shortens the duration or severity of the illness. Acute diarrhoeas most often occur in areas where diagnostic laboratory facilities are limited and treatment, therefore, becomes empirical. Such use of antimicrobial agents is considered hazardous, at best. Injudicious use of antimicrobials involves the risk of the development of resistant strains of pathogens, elimination of normal flora from the intestinal tract and possible toxic side effects of the agent (Gorbach 1982). However, since recent studies have suggested that they may be useful in certain specific infections and in nonspecific therapy of traveller's diarrhoea, we have included a brief section on their use.

The World Health Organization has suggested that there are only four specific indications for the use of antimicrobials in acute diarrhoea: cholera, severe *Shigella* dysentery, amoebic dysentery and acute giardiasis. The recommended treatments for these diseases are given in Table 9.1. Obviously, antimicrobial therapy may also be indicated if the diarrhoea is associated with other acute systemic infections.

Trimethoprim/sulfamethaxazole (TMP/SMX) has recently shown to be effective in the treatment of traveller's diarrhoea caused primarily by enterotoxigenic *E. coli*, and less commonly by *Shigella* and unidentified organisms (DuPont et al 1982). TMP/SMX-treated patients recovered from the diarrhoea significantly faster than untreated patients, 29 hours of illness versus 93 hours in controls, regardless of the aetiologic agent involved. Whereas the results suggest that there may be some value in the use of TMP/SMX for non-specific treatment of acute diarrhoeas, controlled studies would be necessary before this would be recommended. Potential problems also exist, however, since a large number of TMP-resistant bacteria have been isolated from the faeces of treated patients (Murray et al 1982).

Table 9.1 Recommended antimicrobials for enteric infections requiring treatment

Disease	Drug	Adult dose	Children's dose
Cholera	1)[a] Tetracycline	250–500 mg qid × 3–5 days	12 mg/kg qid for 3–5 days
	2)[b] Ampicillin[c]	250 mg qid for 5 days	12–25 mg/kg qid for 5 days
Shigella dysentery	1) Trimethoprim/ sulfamethoxazole	160 mg TMP/800 mg SMX bid for 5 days	5 mg/kg TMP — 25 mg/kg SMX bid for 5 days
	2) Ampicillin[d]	500 mg qid for 5 days	12–25 mg/kg qid for 5 days
Intestinal amoebiasis	1) Metronidazole[e]	750 mg tid for 5–10 days	10 mg/kg tid for 5–10 days
	2) Dehydroemetine hydrochloride	1–1.5 mg/kg IM for 5–10 days	1–1.5 mg/kg IM for 1–5 days
Acute giardiasis	1) Quinacrine	100 mg tid for 5 days	2 mg/kg tid for 5 days (Max. 300 mg/day)
	2) Metronidazole	250 mg tid for 5 days	5 mg/kg tid for 5 days

[a] 1) Indicates drug of choice
[b] 2) Indicates alternative drug
[c] Additional alternatives are: furazolidone, erythromycin, chloramphenicol, doxycycline and trimethoprim/sulfamethoxazole
[d] Additional alternative: tetracycline
[e] Follow metronidazole with di-iodohydroxyquin to remove intraluminal encycsted organisms.

ANTIDIARRHOEAL THERAPY

The long list of potential antidiarrhoeal drugs continues to grow, indicating that no one drug or combination of drugs offers the perfect solution to the problem. While the classical view of diarrhoea pathophysiology has been oriented toward derangements of motility, recent evidence puts emphasis on the importance of abnormalities of intestinal fluid and electrolyte transport, particularly secretion. In light of this, our discussion of the mechanisms of actions of the various antidiarrhoeal agents will focus on the abilities of these agents to alter transport with only a brief review of effects on motility, where appropriate. In order to discuss effectively the antisecretory potential of the antidiarrhoeal drugs it is necessary briefly to review current concepts of fluid and electrolyte transport. This is meant to be only a brief summary and the reader is referred to previous reviews (Powell & Field 1980, Powell 1983, Keusch & Donowitz 1983, Ooms 1983) for a more detailed discussion of this topic.

Pathophysiology

Absorption and secretion are two-part processes: ions enter one cell border, often by carrier mediated processes, and exit the opposite cell border, often by active transport. The direction of fluid movement, into or out of the gut lumen, is an osmotic response to the net movement of electrolytes across the gut mucosa [Figs 9.1(a) and (b)]. Sodium is the ion actively transported during water absorption. Coupled NaCl entry processes on the apical cell membrane increase Na concentrations in the villus cell. The sodium entering with the chloride is transported across the basolateral membrane by NaK-ATPase. Chloride is the ion mediating intestinal secretion. Coupled NaCl entry processes on the basolateral membrane increase the Cl concentration of crypt cells to a level above equilibrium. Therefore, secretory processes are, in some respects, the opposite of absorption. Various secretory stimuli, via intracellular messengers such as cyclic nucleotides and calcium, have two effects: 1) an 'antiabsorptive' action that inhibits NaCl entry across the apical membrane, thus reducing Na and water absorption, and 2) a secretory action through increases in crypt cell apical membrane permeability to Cl, allowing it to leave the cell (be 'secreted'). The two events in concert cause the blood to lumen flow of water.

The major intracellular messengers of stimulus-secretion coupling in the gut are cyclic nucleotides and calcium. Figure 9.1(c) is a schematic representation of the proposed interaction of the intracellular messengers, various secretory stimuli and cellular mechanisms of intestinal ion transport. *E. coli* and cholera enterotoxins stimulte adenylate or guanylate cyclase, increasing intracellular levels of cyclic AMP and cyclic GMP. Prostaglandins and bradykinins are released during inflammation and tissue damage and thus may play an important role in the diarrhoeas due to invasive organisms. The

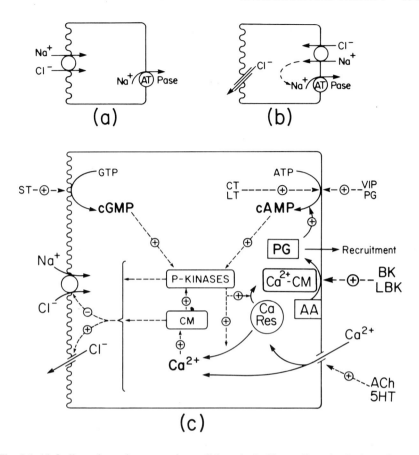

Fig. 9.1 (a) Sodium absorption occurs in small intestinal villous cells and colonic surface cells by virtue of coupled entry across the apical membrane and ATPase mediated exit across the basolateral membrane. Water absorption is an osmotic result of Na absorption. (b) Chloride secretion from small intestinal or colonic crypt cells is the result of changes in apical membrane Cl permeability and egress of Cl from the cell. Coupled NaCl entry mechanisms on the basolateral membranes of these secretory cells allow Cl to reach intracellular concentrations above electrochemical potential. Water secretion will follow the net transport of Cl into the lumen. (c) The three intracellular mediators of intestinal secretion, cyclic GMP, cyclic AMP and Ca^{2+}, are increased by bacterial toxins — *E. coli* heat-stable toxin (ST) and *E. coli* heat-labile toxin (LT), cholera toxin (CT), and by neurohumoral agents — vasoactive intestinal polypeptide (VIP), prostaglandins and leukotrienes (PG), acetylcholine (ACh), serotonin (5HT), bradykinin (BK) or kallidin (LBK). Cyclic nucleotides inhibit coupled NaCl entry or stimulte Cl exit across the apical cell membrane through protein kinases (P-KINASE). Alternatively, cyclic nucloetide-related P-kinases might release ionized calcium (Ca^{2+}) from intracellular reservoirs (Ca Res). Increases in intracellular Ca^{2+} may also inhibit coupled NaCl uptake and promote Cl secretion via calmodulin (CM)-dependent protein kinases. A supplementary action of Ca^{2+}-CM might activate phospholipases releasing arachidonic acid (AA) with the subsequent formation of prostaglandins and leukotrienes. These PG's might stimulate the production of cyclic AMP (or cyclic GMP) in some specific, transport-related cyclic nucleotide pool, could also stimulate adjacent cells to secrete (recruitment), and could modulate intestinal motility and/or blood flow. Ca^{2+}-CM is also a necessary cofactor for cyclic nucleotide synthesis and degradation.

prostaglandins may be also working as intracellular messengers since metabolites of the arachidonic acid cascade may stimulate production of cyclic AMP or cyclic GMP.

Calcium has also been proposed as an important intermediate in secretory diarrhoeas. Calcium may be released from intercellular reservoirs by cyclic nucleotides. Also, agents such as the neurotransmitters acetylcholine (ACh) and serotonin (5-HT) allow calcium 'gating' across the basolateral membrane, thus increasing the ionic concentration of Ca within the cell. The Ca may then stimulate or inhibit Na and Cl transport processes via calcium-calmodulin mediated protein kinases. Cassuto et al (1981) have proposed that bacterial enterotoxins may stimulate release of serotonin from enterochromaffin cells in the gut epithelium. The serotonin might have secretory activity itself or it might release secretory peptides such as vasoactive intestinal polypeptide (VIP) or ACh from mucosal neurons. Thus the schemes of hormone or neurotransmitter-stimulated secretions could be a part of enterotoxin-induced secretion as well.

POTENTIAL ANTIDIARRHOEAL AGENTS

Antidiarrhoeal agents may be categorized according to their mechanism of action. In this section we will first discuss the classic or commercially available agents within a category and then comment on the more experimental drugs in that group.

Luminally active agents

Absorbents, astringents and gels have long been considered useful in the symptomatic relief of diarrhoea. They are believed to act by binding toxins, altering intestinal flora or coating the intestinal mucosa. Little research has documented the efficacy of these agents. Two recent studies involving the popular combination of kaolin and pectin suggest that, while this compound may change stool consistency, it does not alter stool frequency, volume or systemic fluid losses (Portnoy et al 1976, McClung et al 1980) and may actually increase stool sodium and potassium excretion (McClung et al 1980). These results suggest that kaolin-pectin may be useful in the symptomatic relief of mild self-limiting diarrhoea, but should be used with caution in severe diarrhoeas where it may exacerbate electrolyte losses and at the same time mask this effect by changing stool consistency.

Other agents, such as the GM_1 ganglioside bound to charcoal and bile salt binding resins, are being tested as possible means for binding intraluminal enterotoxins. These agents may have significant binding capacity but they appear to have limited clinical effectiveness (McCloy & Hoffman 1971, Stoll et al 1980). They are not capable of reversing the effects of toxin which has already bound to cell membranes, and it may be difficult for them to interact with and neutralize toxin which has been produced by bacteria which adhere to the mucosa (Holmgren & Svennerholm 1982). It is possible that they may be more useful if combined with some kind of anticolonizing therapy.

Astringents are primarily salts of heavy metals such as bismuth, lanthanum and aluminium. Little is known about the specific mechanism of these large polyvalent cations. They will be discussed in the section on calcium/calmodulin.

Antimotility drugs

The belief that diarrhoea was a function of deranged motility resulted in a large number of drugs being proposed as antidiarrhoeal agents based on their ability to influence intestinal muscle function. One group in this class is the anticholinergics whose primary action in the intestinal tract is to inhibit motility. There is little documented research to support the use of anticholinergics in the treatment of diarrhoea; nonetheless, claims of effectiveness still persist (Weiner 1980). A recent study comparing an anticholinergic agent to placebo in relieving traveller's diarrhoea found that there was no improvement in stool consistency, frequency or in the duration of the illness (Reeves et al 1983). Considering the high incidence of undesirable side effects such as headaches, blurred vision, urinary retention and others, along with a very low efficacy, the use of anticholinergic drugs for the treatment of acute diarrhoea is not recommended.

Opiates, the second major group in this class, gained popularity as antidiarrhoeal agents due to their historical efficacy in the empirical treatment of diarrhoea. This category includes natural opiates such as morphine, codeine and paregoric; synthetic opiates such as diphenoxylate and loperamide; and the new peptide opiates such as the enkephalins. All have been shown to have profound effects on gut motility. They increase non-propulsive contractions in the intestinal wall, thereby slowing the flow of intestinal contents and allowing more time for the mucosa to absorb fluid and electrolytes. These actions on gut motility also may contribute to the undesirable effects of opiates including ileus, nausea, delayed gastric emptying and the sequestration of fluid in the intestinal lumen. This group of drugs is also notorious for side effects involving the central nervous system, such as drowsiness, personality changes, respiratory depression, and hypotension, as well as addiction and potential for drug abuse. The effects of opiates on motility were, and, by many, are still believed to be the major mechanism for their antidiarrhoeal activity. Recent studies, however, have demonstrated that the opiates also influence water and electrolyte transport across the intestinal mucosa (Karim & Adaikan 1977, Coupar 1978, Beubler & Lembeck 1979, Dobbins et al 1980, Hardcastle et al 1981, Ilundain & Naftalin 1981, McKay et al 1981, Sandhu et al 1981, Beubler 1982, Hughes et al 1982, McKay et al 1982, Watt et al 1982, Hughes & Turnberg 1982, Turnberg 1983, Sandhu et al 1983). The mechanism by which the opiates exert this influence is not clear. It is not certain whether opiates act on receptors on the enterocytes or whether they act on the enteric nervous system to inhibit the release of secretory transmitters.

Paregoric and deodorized tincture of opium are hydroalcoholic extracts of opium which have been used empirically as antidiarrheal agents for many years. The relatively recent advent of more refined and less complex antidiarrhoeal agents has caused a decline in their usage. They are clinically effective against mild chronic diarrhoea but they are not specific and caution must be exercised to avoid addiction or abuse.

The use of morphine as an antidiarrhoeal agent dates back to the Chinese dynasties. While it is more commonly employed for its analgesic and central nervous system effects, morphine is very effective in inhibiting intestinal secretion and propulsive motility. Besides blocking secretion stimulated by a variety of agents (Coupar 1978, Turnberg 1983), morphine also reduces the intestinal fluid volume in normal subjects (Beubler & Lembeck 1979). Thus, overuse of morphine may result in severe constipation. The central effects of morphine, along with its high abuse potential and addictive properties, make it a poor choice for routine treatment of diarrhoea.

Codeine is an effective antidiarrhoeal agent and has fewer adverse side effects than morphine. Its effects on electrolyte transport are less potent than those of morphine (Racusen et al 1978). One study suggests that, at the doses of the drug that are clinically efficacious, the antidiarrhoeal effect of codeine is due to its antimotility rather than antisecretory properties (Schiller et al 1982). Obviously, the mechanism of antidiarrhoeal action of this and other opiates is still very controversial.

Loperamide is probably the most widely used commercially available antidiarrhoeal agent. Clinically it has been shown to have a more rapid onset of action and require a lower dose than diphenoxylate or morphine for controlling acute diarrhoea (Amery et al 1975, Heel et al 1978). It is better tolerated than other opiates with only mild, transient side effects such as nausea, abdominal pain, dizziness and dry mouth reported in clinical trials with adult patients (Heel et al 1978). Infants and children may be less tolerant. Adverse effects reported include ileus (Sandhu et al 1983b), drowsiness, irritability (Marcovitch 1980) and, in an accidental overdose, a 4-month-old infant exhibited bradypnoea, meiosis and somnolence (Friedli & Haenggeli 1980). The usefulness of this drug in children is not certain. While it has been efficacious in some cases of chronic diarrhea in infants (Sandhu et al 1983b), not all patients respond to the drug and reports on its effectiveness in children with acute diarrhoea are inconclusive (Prakash et al 1980).

Experimental work in laboratory animals and man has shown that loperamide is capable of inhibiting cyclic nucleotide-mediated intestinal secretion stimulated by prostaglandins, bile acids, vasoactive intestinal polypeptide, cholera toxin and heat stable *E. coli* enterotoxin, but it is without effect on calcium-mediated secretion stimulated by carbachol or colchicine. Even though this evidence suggests that loperamide is blocking cyclic nucleotide-mediated secretion, it must do so at some step distal to cyclic nucleotide production because loperamide, as well as many of the other opiates, does not affect the cellular levels of cyclic AMP produced by these various stimuli (Sandhu et al 1981, Farack et al 1981).

Diphenoxylate, the synthetic predecessor to loperamide, has also proven effective as an antidiarrhoeal agent. It is less sepcific for the gut than loperamide. Commercially available in combination with atropine, it can be as effective in controlling diarrhoea as loperamide; however, it requires a higher dose and undesirable side effects are much more common (Avery et al 1975). Because diphenoxylate is given in combination with atropine to reduce the potential for drug abuse, it has all the potential side effects of opiates discussed above as well as those of the anticholinergic agents. This drug, as well as the other antimotility drugs, must be used with caution in the face of potentially invasive aetiologic agents. Diphenoxylate-atropine has been shown to cause a prolonged febrile response in patients with shigellosis (DuPont & Hornick 1973).

The enkephalins are a new group of opiates only recently being explored for treatment of diarrhoea. The endogenous peptide opiates exist naturally in many tissues of the body, including the intestines. They are 10 to 100 times more potent than morphine in altering intestinal transport (McKay et al 1981), potencies that are opposite to those on smooth muscle. Their activity is less well blocked by opiate antagonists such as naloxone and enkephalins originating from gut mucosa tend to have less central effects than other opiates (McKay et al 1981). These differences in action are the result of different opiate receptors located in various parts of the body. The mu (μ)-opiate receptors are located primarily in smooth muscle and they mediate motor function, while the intestinal mucosa contains a high percentage of delta (δ)-receptors which exert a strong influence on intestine electrolyte transport. The high affinity of enkephalins for δ-receptors and morphine for μ-receptors explains their specificities (Chang & Cuatrecasas 1979, Kachur et al 1980, Kachur & Miller 1982). Receptor-specificity is also a potential guide for the production of new more specific antidiarrhoeal agents. Opiates which bind only the receptor controlling intestinal secretion or absorption might have the properties of the 'ideal' antidiarrhoeal agent.

Anti-inflammatory agents

Several of the non-steroidal anti-inflammatory agents have exhibited some degree of antidiarrhoeal activity. The most common of these is aspirin or acetylsalicylic acid (ASA). While the detrimental effects of this drug, including gastrointestinal haemorrhage and exacerbation of gastric acid-peptic disease, have been well documented, the possible beneficial effects of ASA in treating secretory diarrhoeas are less well defined. ASA stimulates Na and Cl absorption in normal rabbit ileum (Powell et al 1979) and inhibits cholera toxin induced secretion in the small intestine (Finck & Katz 1972, Farris et al 1976). Salicyclates have also been shown to decrease the fluid loss of acute diarrhoea in children (Burke et al 1980). The mechanism of ASA's antidiarrhoeal effect is not fully understood. Increased prostaglandin levels cause increased production of cyclic AMP and result in the stimulation of intestinal secretion, so it is possible that inhibition of prostaglandin synthetase is involved in the antisecretory effect of ASA. Alternatively, ASA may inhibit protein kinases or some other step distal to the production of cyclic AMP in the process of intestinal secretion.

In spite of its apparent antisecretory capabilities, aspirin has not yet gained wide acceptance as an antidiarrhoeal agent. This is not true of some of the other salicyclate compounds. Bismuth subsalicylate (Pepto-Bismol®) is a commonly available, well recognized antidiarrhoeal agent which has proven effective in both laboratory animals and man (Goldenberg et al 1975, DuPont et al 1977, Ericsson et al 1977). Its only drawback for clinical use is the volume of the compound that must be given to be effective (DuPont et al 1977). The antidiarrhoeal action of this compound may involve, at least in part, an antisecretory action of the bismuth. However, the salicylate portion of this compound probably plays a significant role in its antidiarrhoeal action.

Sulfasalazine is yet another salicylate compound, currently employed as an anti-inflammatory medication for inflammatory bowel disease (ulcerative colitis and Crohn's colitis), that may have antidiarrhoeal activity. Once in the gut, sulfasalazine is broken down by the intestinal flora to sulfapyradine and 5-amino salicylate. The sulfapyradine is absorbed from the gut and excreted unchanged in the urine with little effect on the intestinal flora. Thus it seems that the anti-inflammatory/anti-diarrhoeal action of sulfasalazine is not due to antimicrobial activity. 5-amino salicylic acid, like the other salicylates, inhibits arachidonic acid metabolism and this process may be involved in its antidiarrhoeal activity. Neither 5-amino salicylic acid nor sulfasalazine have been evaluated for effectiveness in treating acute secretory diarrhoea.

Non-salicylate anti-inflammatory agents have also been found to be useful in blocking stimulated secretion in the intestine. Indomethacin has been shown to be at least partially effective against the enterotoxins of *Vibrio cholerae*, *Shigella flexneri*, and *Salmonella typhimurium* (Smith et al 1981) as well as heat stable *E. coli* enterotoxin (ST) (Greenberg et al 1980). In the ST induced secretion, indomethacin blocked production of cyclic GMP, the agent thought to mediate the secretory process. The usefulness of indomethacin in the treatment of acute diarrhoea is questionable, however, because the inhibitory effects of the drug can be overcome by increasing doses of toxin, suggesting that it may be only marginally effective. Clinical use of indomethacin may be limited by its side effects which include anorexia, nausea, vomiting, peptic ulcers and abdominal pain.

The secretory influence of the prostaglandins and the relative efficacy of some of the prostaglandin inhibitors in controlling diarrhoea raise the possibility that other inhibitors of arachidonic acid metabolism may be useful in the treatment of acute diarrhoea. For instance, the lipoxygenase products of arachidonic acid metabolism, the leukotrienes, have also been implicated in inflammatory and infectious intestinal disease processes. A variety of experimental compounds directed at blocking production of prostaglandins and leukotrienes are being tested in various tissues and animal models. It is possible that we may eventually be able to selectively block the production of 'harmful' arachidonic acid metabolites.

Calcium calmodulin active agents

Calcium and calmodulin have been found to play a significant role in mediating intestinal secretion (Powell & Field 1980, Zimmerman et al 1983). Based on that information, drugs which interact with these two factors would be useful in controlling diarrhoea. The phenothiazine derivatives, notably chlorpromazine (CPZ) and trifluroperazine, have been shown to bind calmodulin and inhibit calmodulin mediated processes. These drugs, originally used for their psychotropic effects, have been shown to possess antisecretory potential as well (Rabbani et al 1979, Holmgren & Greenough 1980, Donowitz et al 1980, Islam et al 1982). They will inhibit in vitro intestinal secretion stimulated by cholera toxin, PGE_2, *E. coli* enterotoxins, cyclic AMP and the calcium ionophore A23187 (Smith & Field 1980). Clinical trials of CPZ against cholera have shown that it significantly reduced fluid losses in patients with high purging rates but no beneficial effect was detectable in the milder cases (Islam et al 1982). The mild sedation and antiemetic action which occurred as a side effect of the CPZ was regarded as favourable in these studies where patients were being rehydrated intravenously (Rabbani et al 1979). This effect is less desirable when depending on oral fluid replacement since sedated patients tend to ingest less fluid. Trifluoperazine has also been shown to be clinical efficacious (Donowitz et al 1980); however, significant side effects, such as postural hypotension, may also make this drug unfavourable for routine use.

Since calcium/calmodulin mediates at least part of the intestinal secretory processes, inhibiting the entry of calcium into cells or binding to cellular proteins may have antisecretory effects. Polyvalent heavy metals such as lanthanum, aluminium and bismuth, may be capable of blocking Ca channels into cells or occupying Ca binding sites on cellular membranes and electrolyte transport-related proteins. Lanthanum has been shown to interfere with Ca-mediated processes in other systems (Greenberg et al 1982) and aluminium hydroxide is commonly used to inhibit secretion by human sweat glands and is quite constipating when given orally. Further study of the potential use for heavy metal compounds as antidiarrhoeal agents is warranted.

Other agents, such as verapamil or nifedipine, which are capable of blocking Ca entry into cells may prove to be useful in inhibiting Ca-mediated secretion. A major pharmacological challenge would be to find a compound which is specific for intestinal epithelial cells since a blockage of Ca entry into other cells produces serious cardiovascular side effects.

Neurotransmitters

Intestinal function, electrolyte transport and motility are controlled in part by the autonomic and enteric nervous systems. Various neurotransmitters, when added exogenously, will stimulate either absorption or secretion of electrolytes and water and will alter motility patterns in the intestine (Racusen & Binder 1979, Weinman et al 1982, Doherty & Hancock 1983). Opposing effects can be demonstrated depending on the type and location of the cellular membrane receptors. Alpha-adrenoreceptor agonists influence both absorptive processes and motility patterns: stimulation of absorption occurs in both the normal and the diarrhoeaic bowel (Doherty & Hancock 1983). Clonidine and lindamine, both alpha-adrenergic agonists, have been shown to have antisecretory effects in laboratory animals (Spraggs & Bunce 1982, Doherty & Hancock 1983) and antidiarrhoeal action in humans (McArthur et al 1982). Clonidine was effective in decreasing stool output in diarrhoea induced by castor oil and by a VIP (vasoactive intestinal polypeptide) producing tumour. While both drugs were effective in suppressing diarrhoea, their potential for use as routine antidiarrhoeal agents is decreased by accompanying side effects such as hypotension, depression and altered levels of glucagon and insulin. These hormonal alterations cause hyperglycaemia and a suppression of the compensatory response to hypoglycaemia. These effects make close monitoring of the patient essential.

The dopaminergic agonists, dopamine and bromocriptine, are related compounds which have been examined for antisecretory activity. These agents stimulate sodium and chloride absorption from the ileum and colon (Donowitz et al 1982, Donowitz et al 1983) via both dopamine and alpha$_2$-adrenergic receptors (Donowitz et al 1983). The clinical usefulness of dopamine is questionable as its effect in vitro is shortlived and the drug cannot be administered orally. Bromocriptine, however, can be given orally, causes prolonged stimulation of dopamine receptors and has been shown to inhibit cholera toxin induced secretion in vitro (Donowitz et al 1982). Again side effects, such as dyspnoea, tachycardia and hypotension, may limit the clinical usefulness of this drug. However, they are reported only evident with initial use and are not so severe as those associated with the strictly alpha$_2$-adrenergic agonists.

Somatostatin is another peptide hormone found in the enteric nervous system which has shown some antidiarrhoeal activity. Besides affecting motility, apparently by inhibiting ACh release, somatostatin inhibits the secretion of a variety of gastrointestinal hormones including gastrin, cholecystokinin, secretin, VIP and GIP (gastrointestinal polypeptide) (Miller et al 1981). It also stimulates absorption of sodium, chloride and bicarbonate and is capable of inhibiting, at least partially, the secretory effects of serotonin and theophylline in vitro (Dobbins et al 1981, Rosenthal et al 1983). The mechanism by which somatostatin mediates these effects is unclear and elucidating it is made even more difficult by the apparent species variation in response to this drug. As with the other drugs in this class, side effects and oral availability limit its usefulness. It would appear that for any of the neurotransmitter type compounds to become effective, clinically useful antidiarrhoeals, new analogues must be found or synthetic modification of the compounds made to improve their specificity.

Miscellaneous

A number of other drugs, which do not neatly fit into the categories discussed above, have been tested or proposed as possible antidiarrhoeal agents. Some have come to attention because of their empirical effect on diarrhoea with no knowledge as to their mechanism of action, others because they theoretically should interfere with some mechanism of secretion which has been identified.

Berberine is a plant alkaloid which has been part of folk medicine in China and India for centuries. Its use in the treatment of diarrhoea came long before any knowledge of mechanisms existed. Recently, both its efficacy and possible mechanisms of action as an antidiarrhoeal have been investigated. Clinical trials have shown that it reduces mortality and shortens the duration of illness in patients with cholera or other non-specific diarrhoeas (Dutta et al 1972, Gaitondé et al 1975). Studies in laboratory animals have demonstrated that berberine is capable of reversing cholera toxin-induced secretion of Na, Cl and water transport in the small intestine; however, it does not affect basal transport (Swabb et al 1981, Tai et al 1981). The mechanism by which it accomplishes this is still unclear: it appears that its site of action may be at some point distal to the production of cyclic AMP or cyclic GMP (Tai et al 1981). From this information it would seem that berberine is close to being the 'ideal' antidiarrhoeal. However, it apparently lacks specificity as it produces a dose-related sedation and hypotension in some species; it is not totally effective in treating human patients, and it also has a very short duration of action (Gaitondé et al 1975, Swabb et al 1981).

Nicotinic acid has also been considered as a possible antidiarrhoeal agent. Information on the antisecretory effects of this compound is rather scarce and somewhat contradictory. In laboratory animals nicotinic acid will reverse cholera toxin-induced fluid accumulation in the rabbit jejunum (Turjman et al 1978, Turjman et al 1980), but it has been observed that fluid accumulation due to cholera toxin is enhanced by nicotinic acid in the rabbit ileum (Gaitondé et al 1975), Clinical trials employing nicotinic acid as an antidiarrhoeal agent have not been reported and its potential for use in this capacity is still unclear.

Serotonin antagonists are potential antidiarrhoeals, but little information is available about the effect of these agents in the gastrointestinal tract. Serotonin (5HT) has been shown to play a role in mediating intestinal secretions, and it is reasonable to expect that an agent which could block cellular 5HT receptors would inhibit secretion stimulated by this means. Unfortunately this is not true for the older and currently available 5HT blockers. While these compounds block 5HT-induced symptoms in the cardiovascular and pulmonary systems, their efficacy in the gastrointestinal tract is minimal. This may be because four different types of 5HT receptors have been identified and the antagonists are being formulated to react with a single species of receptor. It is possible that an antagonist specific for the gastrointestinal mucosa might have useful antisecretory antidiarrhoeal activity.

SUMMARY

The need for a safe, effective antidiarrhoeal agent is clear. Oral rehydration therapy has saved countless lives, but more might survive if secretory rates were diminished simultaneously with this resuscitative therapy. Unfortunately there is no drug currently available which can be uniformly recommended for the routine treatment of acute diarrhoea; their toxic/therapetic ratios have either not been determined or have not proven to be adequate. We have discussed the many agents which are either in use or under study, detailing their efficacy as well as their undesirable side effects. A summary of this information is included in Table 9.2. While it is obvious that further research is necessary, the future is encouraging. As our understanding of the mechanisms controlling intestinal electrolyte transport increases, it is possible that a means to control diarrhoea will become available.

REFERENCES

Amery D, Duyck F, Polak J, Van Den Bouwhuysen G 1975 A multicentre double-blind study in acute diarrhoea comparing Loperamide (R 18553) with two common antidiarrhoeal agents and a placebo. Current Therapy Research 17: 263–270
Beubler E 1983 Anti-secretagogues: therapeutic implications. In: Turnberg L A (ed) Intestinal secretion, BSG:SK & F Work Shop, September 19–21, 1982. Smith, Kline and French Laboratories, Welwyn Garden City, UK
Beubler E, Lembeck F 1979 Inhibition of stimulated fluid secretion in the rat small and large intestine by opiate agonists. Naunyn-Schmiedeberg's Archiv für experimentelle Pathologie u. Pharmakologie 306: 96–98
Black R E, Brown K H, Becker S, Alim A R M A, Huq I 1982 Longitudinal studies of infectious diseases and physical growth of children in rural Bangladesh. II. Incidence of diarrhea and association with known pathogens. American Journal of Epidemiology 115: 315–324
Black R E, Merson M H, Rahman A S M M, Yunus M, Alim A R M A, Huq I, Yolken R H, Curlin G T 1980 A two-year study of bacterial, viral, and parasitic agents associated with diarrhea in rural Bangladesh. Journal of Infectious Diseases 142: 660–664
Burke V, Gracey M, Suharyono, Sunoto 1980 Reduction by aspirin of intestinal fluid-loss in acute childhood gastroenteritis. Lancet i: 1329–1339
Cassuto J, Jodal M, Tuttle R, Lundgren O 1981 On the role of intramural nerves in the pathogenesis of cholera toxin-induced intestinal secretion. Scandinavian Journal of Gastroenterology 16: 377–384

Table 9.2 Summary of the actions of antidiarrhoeal agents

Drug class	Drug	Mechanism of action	Side effects (partial list)
Adsorbents	Kaolin-pectin	Absorbs fluid from luminal contents and changes stool consistency	May increase faecal excretion of sodium and potassium
	GM₁ ganglioside	Binds luminal toxin	
	Cholestyramine	Binds bile acids and possibly luminal enterotoxins	
Anticholinergics		Inhibit intestinal motility	Urinary retention, headaches, blurred vision, etc.
		Block cholinergic 'tone'	
Opiates	DTO	Alter intestinal motility	Respiratory depression, hypotension, ileus, addiction and abuse potential, nausea, vomiting and abdominal pain
	Paregoric	Increase electrolyte absorption	
	Morphine	Cellular mechanisms unknown	
	Codeine		
	Diphenoxylate		
	Loperamide		
	Enkephalins		
Anti-inflammatory agents	Aspirin	Inhibit prostaglandin synthesis	Anorexia, nausea, vomiting, abdominal pain, peptic ulcers, GI bleeding
	Bismuth subsalicylate		
	Sulfasalazine		
	Indomethacin		
Ca/calmodulin	Chlorpromazine	Bind intracellular calmodulin	Cardiovascular abnormalities, i.e. postural hypotension, ventricular arrythmias, heart block, etc.
	Trifluperazine		
	Verapamil	Inhibit Ca entry into cells	
	Nifedipine		
	Lanthanum	Occupy Ca binding sites	
	Aluminium		
	Bismuth		
Neurotransmitters	α-Adrenergics	Stimulate Na and Cl absorption via α₂-adrenergic and dopamine receptors	Hypotension, hyperglycaemia, depression
	clonidine		
	lindamine		
	Dopamine		Dyspnoea, tachycardia, hypotension
	Bromocriptine		
	Somatostatin		

Chang K J, Cuatrecasas P 1979 Multiple opiate receptors. Enkephalins and morphine bind
  to receptors of different specificity. Journal of Biological Chemistry 254: 2610–2618
Coupar I M 1978 Inhibition by morphine of prostaglandin-stimulated fluid secretion in rat
  jejunum. British Journal of Pharmacology 63: 57–63
Dobbins J W, Dharmsathaphorn K, Racusen L, Binder H J 1981 The effect of somatostatin
  and enkephalin on ion transport in the intestine. Annals of the New York Academy of
  Sciences 372: 594–612
Dobbins J, Racusen L, Binder H J 1980 Effect of D-alanine methionine enkephalin amide
  on ion transport in rabbit ileum. Journal of Clinical Investigation 66: 19–28
Doherty N S, Hancock A A 1983 Role of alpha-2 adrenergic receptors in the control of
  diarrhea and intestinal motility. Journal of Pharmacology and Experimental Therapentics
  225: 269–274
Donowitz M, Cusolito S, Battisti L, Fogel R, Sharp G W G 1982 Dopamine stimulation of
  active Na and Cl absorption in rabbit ileum. Journal of Clinical Investigation
  69: 1008–1016
Donowitz M, Elta G, Battisti L, Fogel R, Label-Schwartz E 1983 Effect of dopamine and
  bromocriptine on rat ileal and colonic transport. Gastroenterology 84: 516–23
Donowitz M, Elta G, Bloom S R, Nathanson L 1980 Trifluoperazine reversal of secretory
  diarrhea in pancreatic cholera. Annals of Internal Medicine 93: 284–285
DuPont H L, Hornick R B 1973 Adverse effect of Lomotil therapy in shigellosis. Journal of
  the American Medical Association 226: 1525–1528
DuPont H L, Reves R R, Galindo E, Sullivan P S, Wood L V, Mendiola J G 1982
  Treatment of travelers' diarrhea with trimethoprim/sulfamethoxazole and with
  trimethoprim alone. New England Journal of Medicine 307: 841–844
DuPont, Sullivan P, Pickering L K, Haynes G, Ackerman P B 1977 Symptomatic treatment
  of diarrhea with bismuth subsalicylate among students attending a Mexican university.
  Gastroenterology 73: 715–718
Dutta N K, Marker P H, Rao N R 1972 Berberine in toxin-induced experimental cholera.
  British Journal of Pharmacology 44: 153–159
Ericsson C D, Evans D G, DuPont H L, Evans D J, Pickering L K 1977 Bismuth
  subsalicylate inhibits activity of crude toxins of Escherichia coli and Vibrio cholerae.
  Journal of Infectious Diseases 136: 693–696
Farack U M, Kautz U, Loeschke K 1981 Loperamide reduces the intestinal secretion but
  not the mucosal cAMP accumulation induced by choleratoxin. Naunyn-Schmiedberg's
  Archiv für experimentelle Pathologie u. Pharmakologie 317: 178–179
Farris R K, Tapper E J, Powell D W, Morris S M 1976 Effect of aspirin on normal and
  cholera toxin-stimulated intestinal electrolyte transport. Journal of Clinical Investigation
  57: 916–924
Finck A D, Katz R L 1972 Prevention of cholera-induced intestinal secretion in the cat by
  aspirin. Nature 238: 273–274
Friedli G, Haenggeli C A 1980 Loperamide overdose managed by naloxone. Lancet i: 1413
Gaitondeé B B, Marker P H, Rao N R 1975 Effect of drugs on cholera toxin induced fluid
  in adult rabbit ileal loop. In: Jucken E (ed) Progress in drug research. Birkhauser Verlaz,
  Basel, p 519–526
Goldenberg M M, Honkomp L J, Castellion A W 1975 The antidiarrheal action of bismuth
  subsalicylate in the mouse and the rat. Digestive Diseases 20: 955–960
Gorbach S L 1982 Travelers' diarrhea. New England Journal of Medicine 307: 881–883
Greenberg R N, Murad F, Chang B, Robertson D C, Guerrant R L 1980 Inhibition of
  Escherichia coli heat-stable enterotoxin by indomethacin and chlorpromazine. Infections
  and Immunology 29: 908–913
Greenberg R N, Murad F, Guerrant R L 1982 Lanthanum chloride inhibition of the
  secretory response to Escherichia coli heat-stable enterotoxin. Infections and Immunology
  35: 483–488
Hardcastle J, Hardcastle P T, Read N W, Redfern J S 1981 The action of loperamide in
  inhibiting prostaglandin-induced intestinal secretion in the rat. British Journal of
  Pharmacology 74: 563–569
Heel R C, Brogden R N, Speight T M, Avery G S 1978 Loperamide: a review of its
  pharmacological properties and therapeutic efficacy in diarrhoea. Drugs 15: 33–52
Holmgren J, Greenough W B 1980 Reversal of enterotoxic diarrhea by chlorpromazine and
  related drugs. In: Field M, Fordtran J, Schultz S (eds) Secretory diarrhea. American

Physiological Society, Bethesda, Maryland, ch 16, p 211–218

Holmgren J, Svennerholm A M 1982 Pathogenic mechanisms and new perspectives in the treatment and prevention of enteric infections. Scandinavian Journal of Gastroenterology [Suppl] 77: 47–59

Hughes S, Higgs N B, Turnberg L A 1982 Antidiarrhoeal activity of loperamide: studies of its influence on ion transport across rabbit ileal mucosa in vitro. Gut 23: 974–979

Hughes S, Turnberg L A 1983 Loperamide: in vitro studies of rabbit ileum and in vivo studies in man. In: Turnberg L A (ed) Intestinal secretion, BSG: SK & F Work Shop, September 19–21, 1982. Smith, Kline and French Laboratories, Welwyn Garden City, UK

Islam M R, Sack D A, Holmgren J, Bardhan P K, Rabbani G H 1982 Use of chlorpromazine in the treatment of cholera and other severe acute watery diarrheal diseases. Gastroenterology 82: 1335–1340

Ilundain A, Naftalin R J 1981 The effect of loperamide on cellular control of secretion. Clinical Research Reviews 1 [Suppl 1]: 171–173

Kachur J F, Miller R J 1982 Characterization of the opiate receptor in the guinea-pig ileal mucosa. European Journal of Pharmacology 81: 177–183

Kachur J F, Miller R J, Field M 1980 Control of guinea pig intestinal electrolyte secretion by a δ-opiate receptor. Proceedings of the National Academy of Sciences of the USA 77: 2753–2756

Karim S M M, Adaikan P G 1977 The effect of loperamide on prostaglandin induced diarrhoea in rat and man. Prostaglandins 13: 321–331

Keusch G T, Donowitz M 1983 Pathophysiological mechanisms of diarrhoeal diseases: diverse aetiologies and common mechanisms. Scandinavian Journal of Gastroenterology 18 [Suppl 84]:33–43

Mareovitch H 1980 Loperamide in 'toddler diarrhoea'. Lancet i: 1413

McArthur K E, Anderson D S, Durbin T E, Orloff M J, Dharmsathaphorn K 1982 Clonidine and idamidine to inhibit watery diarrhea in a patients with lung cancer. Annals of Internal Medicine 96: 323–325

McCloy R M, Hofmann A F 1971 Tropical diarrhea in Vietnam — a controlled study of cholestyramine therapy. New England Journal of Medicine 284: 139–140

McClung H J, Beck R D, Powers P 1980 The effect of kaolin-pectin adsorbent on stool losses of sodium, potassium, and fat during a lactose-intolerance diarrhea in rats. Journal of Pediatrics 96: 769–771

McKay J S, Linaker B D, Higgs N B, Turnberg L A 1982 Studies of the antisecretory activity of morphine in rabbit ileum in vitro. Gastroenterology 82: 243–247

McKay J S, Linaker B D, Turnberg L A 1981 Influence of opiates on ion transport across rabbit ileal mucosa. Gastroenterology 80: 279–84

Miller R J, Kachur J F, Field M 1981 Neurohumoral control of ileal electrolyte transport. Annals of the New York Academy of Sciences 571–593

Murray B E, Rensimer E R, DuPont H L 1982 Emergence of high-level trimethoprim resistance in fecal *Escherichia coli* during oral administration of trimethoprim or trimethoprim-sulfamethoxazole. New England Journal of Medicine 306: 130–135

Ooms L 1983 Alterations in intestinal fluid movement. Scandinavian Journal of Gastroenterology 18 [Suppl 84]: 65–77

Portnoy B L, DuPont H L, Pruitt D, Abdo J A, Rodriguez J T 1976 Antidiarrheal agents in the treatment of acute diarrhea in children. Journal of the American Medical Association 236: 844–846

Powell D W Enterotoxigenic diarrhea: mechanisms and prospects for therapy. In: Dorner F, Drews J (eds) The international encyclopedia of pharmacology and therapeutics, 'Pharmacology of bacterial toxins'. Pergamon Press Ltd, in press

Powell D W, Field M 1980 Pharmacological approaches to treatment of secretory diarrhea. In: Field M, Fordtran J, Schultz S (eds) Secretory diarrhea. American Physiological Society, Bethesda, Maryland, ch 16, p 187–209

Powell D W, Tapper E J, Morris S M 1979 Aspirin-stimulated intestinal electrolyte transport in rabbit ileum in vitro. Gastroenterology 74: 1429–1437

Prakash P, Sexena S, Sareen D K 1980 Loperamide versus diphenoxylate in diarrhea of infants and children. Indian Journal of Pediatrics 47: 303–306

Rabbani G H, Holmgren J, Greenough W B, Lonnroth I 1979 Chlorpromazine reduces fluid-loss in cholera. Lancet i: 412

Racusen L C, Binder H J 1979 Adrenergic interaction with ion transport across colonic mucosa: role of both alpha and beta adrenergic agonists. In: Binder H J (ed) Mechanisms of intestinal secretion. Alan R Liss Inc, New York, ch 16, p 201–215

Racusen L C, Binder H J, Dobbins J W 1978 Effects of exogenous and endogenous opiate compounds on ion transport in rabbit ileum in vitro. (Abstract) Gastroenterology 74: 1081

Reves R, Bass P, DuPont H L, Sullivan P, Mendiola J 1983 Failure to demonstrate effectiveness of an anticholinergic drug in the symptomatic treatment of acute travelers' diarrhea. Journal of Clinical Gastroenterology 5: 223–227

Rosenthal L E, Pressman J, Dharmsathaphorn K 1983 Development of new antidiarrheal medications. Journal of Clinical Gastroenterology 5: 131–135

Sandhu B K, Milla P J, Harries J T 1983a Mechanisms of action of loperamide. Scandinavian Journal of Gastroenterology 18 [Suppl 84]: 85–92

Sandhu B K, Tripp J H, Candy D C A, Harries J T 1981 Loperamide: studies on its mechanism of action. Gut 22: 658–662

Sandhu B K, Tripp J H, Milla P J, Harries J T 1983b Loperamide in severe protracted diarrhoea. Archives of Disease in Childhood 58: 39–43

Schiller L R, Davis G R, Santa Ana C A, Morawski S G, Fordtran J S 1982 Studies of the mechanism of the antidiarrheal effect of codeine. Journal of Clinical Investigation 70: 999–1008

Smith P L, Blumberg J B, Stoff J S, Field M 1981 Antisecretory effects of indomethacin on rabbit ileal mucosa in vitro. Gastroenterology 80: 356–65

Smith P L, Field M 1980 In vitro antisecretory effects of trifluoperazine and other neuroleptics in rabbit and human small intestine. Gastroenterology 78: 1545–1553

Spraggs C F, Bunce K T 1983 Alpha 2-adrenoceptors and the delay of castor oil-induced diarrhoea by clonidine in rats. Journal of Pharmacy and Pharmacology 35: 321–322

Stoll B J, Bardhan P K, Greenough W B, Holmgren J, Huq I, Fredman P, Svennerholm L 1980 Binding of intraluminal toxin in cholera: trial of GMI ganglioside charcoal. Lancet ii: 887–891

Swabb E A, Tai Y H, Jordan L 1981 Reversal of cholera toxin-induced secretion in rat ileum by luminal berberine. American Journal of Physiology 241 [Gastrointertinal Liver Physiology 4]: G248–G252

Tai Y H, Feser J F, Marnane W G, Desjeux J F 1981 Antisecretory effects of berberine in rat ileum. American Journal of Physiology 241 [Gastrointestinal Liver Physiology 4]: G253–G258

Turjman N, Cardamone A, Gotterer G S, Hendrix T R 1980 Effect of nicotinic acid on cholera-induced fluid movement and unidirectional sodium fluxes in rabbit jejunum. Johns Hopkins Medical Journal 147: 209–211

Turjman N, Gotterer G S, Hendrix T R 1978 Prevention and reversal of cholera enterotoxin effects in rabbit jejunum by nicotinic acid. Journal of Clinical Investigation 61: 1155–1160

Turnberg L A 1983 Antisecretory activity of opiates in vitro and in vivo in man. Scandinavian Journal of Gastroenterology 18 [Suppl 84]: 79–83

Watt J, Candy D C A, Gregory B, Tripp J H, Harries J T 1982 Loperamide modifies Escherichia coli, heat-stable enterotoxin-induced intestinal secretion. Journal of Pediatric Gastroenterology and Nutrition 1: 583–586

Weiner N 1980 Atropine, scopalamine and related antimuscarinic drugs. In: Gilman A G, Goodman L S, Gilman A (eds) The pharmacological basis of therapeutics, 6th edn. McMillan Publishing Co, New York, ch 7, p 120–137

Weinman E J, Sansom S C, Knight T F, Senekijian H O 1982 Alpha and beta adrenergic agonists stimulate water absorption in the rat proximal tubule. Journal of Membrane Biology 69: 107–111

Zimmerman T W, Dobbins J W, Binder H J 1983 Role of calcium in the regulation of colonic secretion in the rat. American Journal of Physiology 244 [Gastrointestinal Liver Physiology 7]: G552–G560

Oral rehydration therapy — physiological basis

INTRODUCTION

Glucose-linked enhanced sodium and water absorption from the small intestinal lumen is largely intact during acute diarrhoea of diverse aetiology and forms the scientific basis of oral rehydration therapy (ORT). The first deliberate application of this knowledge was made by Phillips (1964) in a few profusely purging adults with cholera in whom an orally administered glucose containing electrolyte solution induced absorption of sodium and water from the small bowel lumen leading to a net positive balance. This demonstration may be regarded as the beginning of the scientific development of oral rehydration therapy. Soon after, a series of careful clinical and metabolic balance studies established the practical usefulness of ORT in adults and children with acute diarrhoea of diverse aetiology. ORT has now emerged as a powerful therapeutic tool and is capable of replacing the need for intravenous rehydration in 80 to 90 per cent of those clinically dehydrated patients with acute diarrhoea who would have received intravenous therapy by hitherto accepted therapeutic criteria.

An impressive demonstration of the practical effectiveness of ORT under the most adverse conditions was during a cholera epidemic among the West Bengal refugee camps during the 1971 Bangladesh war (Mahalanabis et al 1973). This helped to convince the health planners and public health workers of its important role as a health weapon. ORT has now been recognized as one of the few technically simple and widely applicable therapeutic interventions which can substantially reduce mortality from diarrhoea in infants and children. It has been identified by the World Health Organization as an eminently suitable tool for use at the primary health care level and an excellent entry point for appropriate health education activities.

Intestinal absorption

This is a two-stage process; ions enter the enterocyte through the luminal surface usually by a carrier mediated process, and exit through the basolateral membrane, usually by an active transport into the intercellular and

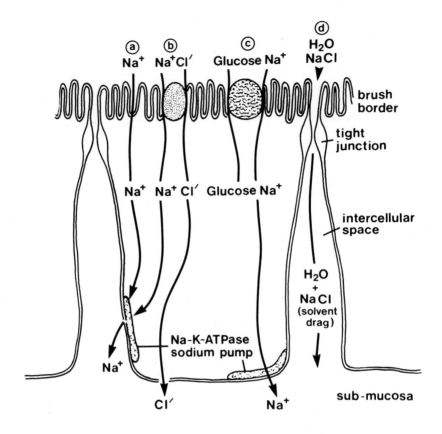

@ⓑ and ⓒ are Transcellular Transport Mechanisms
ⓓ is a Paracellular Transport Mechanism

Fig. 10.1 Water and electrolyte transport and villi enterocytes.

subcellular space. Sodium transport is the primary event during water absorption (see Fig. 10.1). Sodium enters the epithelial cells by three postulated mechanisms.

1. Electroneutral cotransport of Na^+ with Cl^- (Fig. 10.1b). Probably sodium and chloride are not directly coupled but this represents the net result of a double exchange process across the apical membrane whereby Na^+ entry is coupled to H^+ exit, and Cl^- entry is coupled to OH^- (or HCO_3^-) exit. This mechanism probably represents an important method of sodium and chloride absorption from the small bowel under physiological conditions. It is inhibited by cholera toxin and other enterotoxins responsible for secretory diarrhoea.

2. Positive Na^+ diffusion down its electochemical gradient drives this uncoupled electrogenic absorption (Fig. 10.1a) (Schultz 1977). Chlorine ion

is believed to traverse through the tight junction between enterocytes into intercellular space to maintain electrical neutrality.

3. Sodium cotransport coupled to organic solutes such as glucose or amino-acids (Fig. 10.1c). The addition of glucose to solutions in the small intestinal lumen stimulates sodium and water absorption at a substantially enhanced rate over the basal level. The Na^+-glucose coupled entry process results in bulk flow of water both between and through the cells which traps additional sodium and chloride molecules in the flowing stream, the 'solvent drag action'. This glucose-mediated enhancement of sodium and water absorption is the principle behind the sugar substrates in oral rehydration fluids.

The second stage of Na^+ transfer is the active extrusion from the enterocyte by NaK-ATPase, the 'sodium pump' on the basolateral membrane. This leads to a high level of Na^+ in the extracellular spaces with osmotic and hydrostatic effects that increase water absorption.

Intestinal secretion

The secretory process is visualized as the opposite of absorption. The coupled sodium-chloride entry process on the basolateral membrane increases the Cl^- concentration within the crypt cells to a level above the electrochemical equilibrium, while sodium is actively extruded back across the basolateral membrane by the NaK-ATPase into intercellular space (Fig. 10.2). Various secretory stimuli, via intracellular messengers such as cyclic nucleotides and calcium, increase the crypt cell apical membrane permeability to chloride, allowing it to be 'secreted'. This movement of chloride and the sodium that accompanies it, creates a blood to lumen flow of water.

The phenomenon of glucose-linked enhanced sodium absorption and its application in ORT

Normal physiology and glucose-linked sodium absorption

In 1902 Waymouth Reid from Scotland, using dog intestinal loops (in vivo), demonstrated enhanced sodium absorption in the presence of glucose by mammalian small intestine (Reid 1902). This phenomenon was confirmed in 1939 by Barany & Sperber (1939). (In vitro studies by Riklis & Quastel (1958) showed that the sodium ion was linked to glucose absorption. Many physiological experiments looked at this phenomenon in the reverse sequence, i.e. dependence of glucose absorption on sodium ions, and these have been reviewed (Czaky, 1963, Crane 1965). However, stimulation of sodium absorption across the small intestinal mucosa by glucose was also looked at by physiologists (Schultz & Zalunsky 1964, Barry et al 1965.) In 1963 Schedl & Clifton (1963), using transintestinal intubation tech-

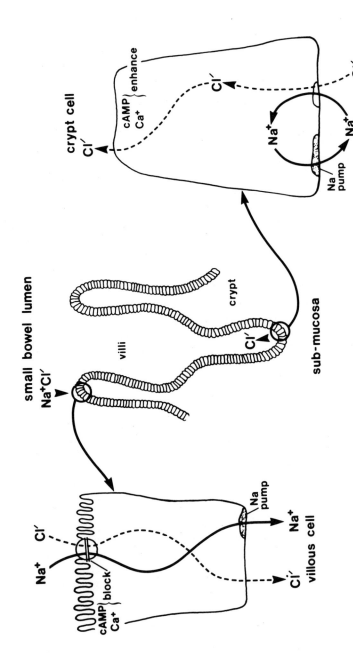

Fig. 10.2 Na⁺ and Cl⁻ small bowel absorption and secretion.

niques in human volunteers, demonstrated a dramatic improvement in sodium chloride and water absorption from Ringer's solution in both the jejunum and ileum by adding 1 g per 100 ml glucose. Subsequent in vivo studies in normal human small intestine defined the quantitative relationships of glucose linked enhanced sodium and water absorption (Malawar et al 1965, Levinson & Schedl 1966, Fordtran et al 1968).

Glucose-linked sodium absorption during acute diarrhoeal illness

In 1964 Robert Phillips, a student of Van Slyke, studied the effect of orally administered glucose-containing electrolyte solution on the net intestinal balance in a few actively purging cholera patients. In this classical model of watery diarrhoea he demonstrated a positive balance for sodium and water absorption over a short period of time, having failed to do so on earlier occasions using a glucose-free electrolyte solution (Phillips 1964). This is probably the first documented evidence that this glucose-linked sodium absorption is largely unaffected during an acute diarrhoeal illness. Independent studies from Calcutta (Pierce et al 1968a, 1968b, 1969) and Dhaka (Hirschhorn et al 1968, Nalin et al 1968) provided more definitive evidence that during the phase of active purging in adult cholera patients fluid and electrolyte losses were adequately replaced by optimally constituted oral electrolyte solution containing glucose. Radioactive tracer studies in cholera patients also showed that 2 g per 100 ml glucose induced net absorption of sodium and water from the small intestine (Taylor et al 1968). Carpenter et al (1968) confirmed this phenomenon experimentally by showing that in the canine jejunal and ileal Thiry-Vella loops challenged with crude cholera toxin, net sodium and water loss was reduced when glucose was added to the perfusion electrolyte solution.

Glucose-linked sodium absorption and experience with ORT

The initial success of ORT in adult cholera patients was tested by its vigorous application (under controlled conditions) in treating diarrhoeal disease in children with cholera, in infants and small children with diarrhoea induced by rotavirus, enterotoxigenic *E. coli* and other aetiological agents. It emerged as a powerful therapeutic tool with the ability to correct dehydration due to acute diarrhoea in all but the most severe cases, and in all ages irrespective of aetiological agents (Mahalanabis 1984, WHO 1983).

ORAL REHYDRATION FLUIDS

An orally administered solution for the treatment of acute diarrhoea should optimally meet the conditions that govern net absorption of electrolytes and water by the intestine, and at the same time fulfil the need of fluid therapy in acute diarrhoeal illness.

Components of an oral rehydration solution, physiology of intestinal absorption and the therapeutic need in acute diarrhoea

Sodium

Substantial sodium loss occurs in diarrhoeal dehydration. A child with moderate to severe dehydration due to acute diarrhoea may lose 8–12 mmol of sodium associated with an average water loss of 100 ml for each kilogram of body weight (10 per cent of body weight). As stated earlier, the jejunum and ileum absorb sodium at an enhanced rate in the presence of glucose, and the nearer the luminal sodium concentration is to the plasma level, the better its net absorption (Sladen & Dawson 1969). Water is absorbed passively in the direction of the osmotic flow. Perfusion studies in human volunteers using short jejunal segments showed that net sodium absorption from an iso-osmotic glucose electrolyte solution drops to zero when its concentration is brought down from 105 to 77 mmol per litre. When extrapolated to an intact animal situation, net absorption of glucose and water should only take place from such a solution until its sodium concentration reaches a high enough level for its absorption to occur. Sodium absorption is also augmented by bicarbonate independently of glucose (see below).

Chloride

Loss of chloride in diarrhoeal dehydration is closely linked to sodium loss and is of the same order of magnitude, its absorption being closely linked to sodium absorption.

Potassium

The magnitude of potassium loss in diarrhoeal dehydration in infants and children can be as high as that of sodium. Potassium is lost both in the stool as well as in the urine during the development of dehydration. Potassium losses in acute diarrhoea can be particularly harmful in infants, especially those that are undernourished and therefore relatively depleted from the start. Potassium absorption takes place passively depending on the concentration gradient. Thus, a luminal potassium concentration higher than that in plasma will induce absorption which is independent of glucose absorption. The potassium concentration of 20 mmol/litre of standard oral rehydration formulations is well tolerated and helps replacement therapy. However, additional potassium containing food and drinks during and after diarrhoea are required for adequate replacement of potassium deficit.

Bicarbonate

Varying degrees of base deficit acidosis occurs in diarrhoeal dehydration. Bicarbonate in oral rehydration solution, as $NaHCO_3$, helps to correct acidosis faster than in its absence. Bicarbonate is actively absorbed from the jejunum against a steep electrochemical gradient and enhances sodium absorption independently (Turnberg et al 1970a, 1970b, Fordtran et al 1968), even when glucose-linked enhanced sodium absorption is maximized (Mahalanabis & Patra 1983).

Osmolality

In the duodenum and jejunum isotonic osmolality is quickly attained in ingested fluid by the flow of water and/or solutes. Hence, intake of an iso-osmotic oral rehydration fluid should create minimal disequilibrium (Fordtran et al 1966, Sladen & Dawson 1969). Solutions rendered hyperosmolar with high concentrations of glucose and/or other sugars may lead to incomplete absorption and osmotic watery diarrhoea (see below).

Glucose and its substitutes

A glucose concentration in the range of 20–30 g per litre of oral rehydration formulations stimulates optimum absorption except in a very small proportion of clinically dehydrated hospitalized patients who may develop temporary glucose malabsorption. Higher concentrations of glucose (e.g. 40 g per litre) may lead to its incomplete absorption and osmotic diarrhoea in a large proportion of patients.

Sucrose is an adequate alternative to glucose when approximately twice the amount is used in oral rehydration formulations (e.g. 40 g sucrose in place of 20 g glucose per litre). A slightly higher failure rate of sucrose containing formulations may be related to slow absorption of fructose liberated from hydrolysis of sucrose creating adverse osmotic effects.

Recently, oral rehydration formulations containing 30–50 g cooked rice powder (Molla et al 1982, Patra et al 1982) in place of glucose have been found to be highly effective (see below). Rice, on digestion, should yield glucose, amino acids and small peptides all of which can stimulate sodium absorption.

Finally, oral rehydration formulations containing both glucose and an amino acid glycine (Patra et al 1984) have been shown to be even more efficient than standard glucose-based oral rehydration formulations (see below).

Oral rehydration formulations

Universal oral rehydration formulation recommended by WHO/UNICEF

Based on principles discussed, WHO has recommended, since 1971, an oral rehydration formulation to treat dehydration from diarrhoea of any cause, including cholera, in all age groups. It has the following composition:

Sodium chloride	3.5 grams
Sodium hydrogen carbonate (Sodium bicarbonate)	2.5 grams
Potassium chloride	1.5 grams
Glucose	20.0 grams

To be dissolved in one litre of clean drinking water.

This formulation is generally provided prepacked in a dry form called ORS to be reconstituted when required. These ingredients are distributed by UNICEF in aluminium foil packets labelled 'Oral Rehydration Salts'. This complete WHO-recommended formula is regarded as the most physiologically appropriate single formulation for worldwide use. ORS, when reconstituted, has the following composition:

Sodium	90 mmol/litre
Potassium	20 mmol/litre
Chloride	80 mmol/litre
Bicarbonate	30 mmol/litre
Glucose	111 mmol/litre

From the outset, ORS was envisaged for use both to correct dehydration (the rehydration phase) and to maintain hydration during continuing diarrhoea (the maintenance phase). Extensive experience has repeatedly demonstrated the safety and efficacy of ORS as a universal ORT solution when used correctly (see WHO 1983).

Use of ORS in diarrhoea

A great deal of experience has been gained in the use of ORS for the treatment of dehydration in hospitals, clinics, and homes, both for infants as well as for adults and older children with acute diarrhoea of diverse aetiologies. The composition of ORS (particularly its sodium concentration) is optimal for *rehydration*, i.e. replacement of salt and water deficit that has already occurred in a dehydrated child (Darrow 1946, Darrow et al 1949, Mahalanabis 1970). ORS has also been found to be eminently suitable for the replacement of ongoing diarrhoeal stool losses in infants (including neonates) during *maintenance* therapy, provided their additional water need is met by unrestricted breastfeeding, and in non-breastfed infants giving water, dilute feeds and other fluid drinks after initial rehydration (WHO 1983).

Formulations with lower sodium concentrations can be used for treating most cases of diarrhoea in infants (Chatterjee et al 1977, Chatterjee et al 1978, Santosham et al 1982) they are not, however, suitable for use in patients with cholera and similar secretory diarrhoea.

TREATMENT PRINCIPLES AND OPTIMUM USE OF ORT

It is useful to consider the fluids administered to a dehydrated patient during management of acute diarrhoea as meeting the following essential needs:

(1) *rehydration therapy* — correction of existing water and electrolyte deficit as indicated by the signs of dehydration; (2) *maintenance therapy* — replacement of ongoing abnormal losses of water and electrolytes due to continuing diarrhoea till diarrhoea stops; and (3) provision of daily fluid requirements during rehydration and maintenance, particularly in infants.

Rehydration therapy

This can usually be achieved orally with ORS solution, except in cases with severe dehydration, uncontrollable vomiting or a serious complication that prevents successful oral therapy. An infant with unequivocal signs of dehydration may initially need an average amount of 100 ml per kilogram body weight of ORS solution; this amount can usually be administered in 4 to 6 hours. Larger amounts may be required in some patients while in others smaller quantities may suffice; *the needed amount can be judged adequately by the clinical response.*

Maintenance therapy

After the initial fluid and electrolyte deficit has been corrected, the ongoing abnormal losses due to continuing diarrhoea are replaced by giving appropriate amounts of ORS solution. If the diarrhoea is severe then ORS solution is given at an average rate of 10 to 15 ml per kilogram body weight per hour. In most patients, however, diarrhoeal stool loss is mild to moderate and they are either given (a) ORS solution 100 ml per kilogram per day till diarrhoea stops, or (b) 10 ml ORS solution per kilogram body weight for each diarrhoea stool.

Normal daily fluid requirement

This is particularly important in infants. Breast milk optimally meets this requirement as it is very low in renal solute load, and breastfeeding should be commenced during *rehydration* and continued, unrestricted, during maintenance. In non-breastfed infants plain water (a minimum volume equal to half the amount of ORS solution already taken by the infant) should be given as soon as he is fully rehydrated (usually over 2–3 hours); they should also be offered half-strength formula milk at 3–4 hourly feeds. Other traditional fluids appropriate for age (e.g. rice water, carrot soup or weak tea) may also fulfill this need and are recommended.

Administration of ORS solution

The solution is given to infants using a cup and spoon, a cup alone, or a feeding bottle if he is used to one. For weak, small babies, a dropper or a syringe can be used to put small volumes of solution at a time into the mouth. For babies who cannot drink due to fatigue or drowsiness, but are not in shock, a nasogastric tube can be used to administer the solution; a rate of 15–20 ml per kilogram per hour is well tolerated. *Vomiting* is not uncommon during the first hour or two of administration of ORS solution but it does not usually prevent successful oral rehydration.

Maintenance of nutrition: dietetic management

There is no physiological basis for 'resting' the bowel during or following acute diarrhoea. Fasting has been shown to reduce further the ability of the small intestine to absorb a variety of nutrients. Even during acute diarrhoea a substantial amount of nutrients is absorbed when food is offered. As soon as their appetite returns all children aged 4 months and older should eat semisolid and solid foods; food should be started during maintenance therapy — there is no basis for delay in feeding until diarrhoea stops (Mahalanabis 1983, Molla et al 1983).

SOME ASSOCIATED PROBLEMS AND COMPLICATIONS, AND USE OF ORT

Infants with hypernatraemic dehydration

The WHO-recommended ORS solution has met with uniform success in treating infants with hypernatraemic dehydration. Well over 100 infants (about a quarter of whom were neonates) with hypernatraemic dehydration have been successfully treated, and with excellent results, using ORS. These results appear to be more favourable compared to the best clinical results reported with intravenous therapy (Mahalanabis 1984, Pizarro et al 1984).

Severe malnutrition and ORT

Dehydration due to acute diarrhoea in children with severe protein-energy malnutrition (e.g. marasmus, kwashiorkor) has been managed with ORS solution in the same way as above. In children with kwashiorkor rehydration therapy may increase oedema and the risk of congestive heart failure (as it is with I.V. therapy) and thus should be closely supervized.

Use of ORT in hospitals

Investigations conducted by the Diarrhoeal Diseases Control Programme of WHO revealed that in several major hospitals in the developing countries, successful introduction of oral rehydration therapy with ORS solution has led to a substantial reduction in the cost of treatment due to a large decrease in the use of I.V. fluid and giving sets, and in the number of hospital admissions (as a result of introducing outpatient based oral rehydration therapy programmes); in some hospitals the use of ORS has also resulted in a substantial decrease in the number of deaths from diarrhoea probably due to an overall concern regarding diarrhoea management and a decline in the complications of I.V. therapy.

FUTURE OF ORT

Oral rehydration solution as an absorption promoting drug

ORS, though a powerful therapeutic tool, neither reduces nor increases the magnitude and duration of diarrhoea in infants and children with rotavirus diarrhoea or cholera compared to I.V. treated controls. In adults with cholera diarrhoeal stool output may even increase by about 15 per cent as a result of ORT (Mahalanabis & Patra 1983).

Since almost all water-soluble organic molecules (nutrients being of particular relevance) such as D-hexoses, amino acids, dipeptides and tripeptides, can enhance the absorption of sodium (water absorption being solely dictated by osmotic forces) it is postulated that their optimum combination can effect reabsorption of secreted sodium and water into the small bowel lumen in addition to the absorption of ingested ones and reduce the magnitude and duration of diarrhoea and thus act like an absorption promoting drug. Two recent studies (Patra et al 1982, Patra et al 1984) on infants and small children with acute diarrhoea and moderate to severe dehydration demonstrated that (a) adding the amino acid, glycine, to ORS solution and (b) replacing the 20 g glucose in the ORS formulation by 50 g cooked rice powder lead to a reduction in the diarrhoea stool volume by 50 per cent and in duration of diarrhoea as well as the volume of oral rehydration solution required by 30 per cent. Human perfusion studies showed that dipeptides and tripeptides are absorbed at about 70 per cent faster rate than their constituent amino acids, their absorption is uniformly high in the whole length of the small intestine, their absorption is more robust in disease states and low pH conditions. It is postulated that optimum use of small peptides and their precursors, and D-hexoses and their precursors may further enhance absorption efficiency of ORS, making antidiarrhoeal drugs redundant (Mahalanabis & Patra 1983).

A more stable ORS formulation

In view of the short shelf-life of the present formulation, several studies are being conducted with an ORS formulation in which sodium bicarbonate has been replaced by sodium citrate. Preliminary results suggest that citrate based ORS is as effective as standard ORS.

Cereal-based ORS

Some recent studies (Molla et al, unpublished) showed that further increasing the rice cereal in ORS does not improve absorption efficiency any further. One other study (Patra et al, unpublished) in infantile diarrhoea with glycine-fortified rice-based ORS could not show any further improvement in ORS. The constraints of cereal based ORS include (a) need for cooking prior to use, (b) fermentation and bacterial overgrowth once the solution is made up within a short time, (c) difficulty in making a ready to use packaged product, and (d) incomplete digestion of starch in very young infants. Other cereals are being tested for their efficacy as replacements of glucose in ORS. Defining the role of various cereals in oral rehydration therapy should substantially improve home therapy of diarrhoea and may even decrease the number of referrals to treatment centres. Use of cereals in ORS also assists nutrition therapy of acute diarrhoea.

REFERENCES

Barany E H, Sperber E 1939 Absorption of glucose against a concentration gradient by the small intestine of the rabbit. Scandinavian Archives of Physiology 81–290
Barry R J C, Smyth D H, Wright E M 1965 Short circuit current and solute transfer by rat jejunum. Journal of Physiology 181: 410–431
Carpenter C C J, Sack R B, Feeley J C, Steenberg R W 1968 Site and characteristics of electrolyte loss and effects of intraluminal glucose in experimental canine cholera. Journal of Clinical Investigation 47: 1210–1220
Chatterjee A, Mahalanabis D, Jalan K N et al. Evaluation of a sucrose/electrolyte solution for oral rehydration in acute infantile diarrhoea. Lancet i: 1333–35
Chatterjee A, Mahalanabis D, Jalan K N, Maitra T K, Agarwa S K, Dutta et al 1978 Oral rehydration in infantile diarrhoea. Archives of Disease in Childhood 54: 284–289
Crane R K 1965 Sodium dependent transport in the intestine and other animal tissues Federation Proceedings 24: 1000–1006
Czaky T Z 1963 A possible link between active transport of electrolytes and non-electrolytes. Federation Proceedings 22: 3–7
Darrow D C 1946 The retention of electrolyte during recovery from severe dehydration due to diarrhea. Journal of Pediatrics 28: 515
Darrow D C, Pratt E L, Flett, J Jr, Gamble A H, Wiese H F 1949 Disturbances of water and electrolytes in infantile diarrhea. Pediatrics 3: 129
Fordtran J S, Locklear T W 1966 Ionic consittuents and osmolality of gastric and small-intestinal fluids after eating. American Journal of Digestive Diseases 11(7): 503–521
Fordtran J S, Rector F C, Carter N W 1968 The mechanism of sodium absorption in the human small intestine. Journal of Clinical Investigation 47: 884–900
Hirschhorn H, Kinzie J L, Sechar D B, Northrup R S, Taylor J O, Ahmad S Z et al 1968. Decrease in net stool output in cholera during intestinal perfusion with glucose-containing solutions. New England Journal of Medicine 279: 176–181
Levinson R A, Schedl H P 1966 Absorption of sodium, chloride, water, and simple sugars in rat small intestine. American Journal of Physiology 211: 939–942
Mahalanabis D 1983 Feeding practices in relation to childhood diarrhea and malnutrition. In: Chen L C, Scrimshaw N S (eds) Diarrhea and malnutrition, interactions, mechanisms and interpretations. Plenum Press, NY, p 223–234
Mahalanabis D 1984 In: Chandra R K (ed) Oral rehydration therapy. Critical reviews in tropical medicine. Plenum Press, NY, vol 2, p 77–91
Mahalanabis D, Patra F C 1983 In search of a super oral rehydration solution: Can optimum use of organic solute-mediated sodium absorption lead to the development of an absorption promoting drug? Journal of Diarrhoeal Disease Research 1(2): 76–81
Mahalanabis D, Choudhuri A B, Bagchi N G, Bhattacharya A K, Simpson T W 1973 Oral fluid therapy of cholera among Bangladesh refugees. Johns Hopkins Medical Journal 132(4): 197–205
Mahalanabis D, Wallace C K, Kallen R J, Mondal A, Pierce N F 1970 Water and

electrolyte losses dur to cholera in infants and small children: A recovery balance study. Pediatrics 45: 374

Malawar S J, Enton M, Fordtran J S, Ingelfinger F J 1965 Interrelation between jejunal absorption of sodium glucose and water in man. Journal of Clinical Investigation (Abstract) 44(6): 1072

Molla A, Molla A M, Sarkar S A, Khatoon M, Rahaman M M 1983 Effects of acute diarrhoea on absorption of macronutrients during disease and after recovery. In: Chen L C, Scrimshaw N S (eds) Diarrhoea and malnutrition, interactions, mechanisms and interpretations. Plenum Press, NY, p 143–154

Molla A M, Sarkar S A, Hossain M, Molla A, Greenough W B III 1982 Rice-powder electrolyte solution as oral therapy in diarrhoea due to *Vibrio cholerae* and *Escherichis coli*. Lancet: 1317–19

Nalin D R, Cash R A, Islam R, Molla M, Phillips R A 1968 Oral maintenance therapy for cholera in adults. Lancet: 370–373

Patra F C, Mahalanabis D, Jalan K N, Sen A, Banerjee P 1982 Is oral rice electrolyte solution superior to glucose electrolyte solution in infantile diarrhoea? Archives of Disease in Childhood 57: 910–12

Patra F C, Mahalanabis D, Jalan K L, Sen A, Banerjee P 1984 In search of a super solution: controlled trial of glycine-glucose oral rehydration solution in infantile diarrhoea. Acta Paediatrica Scandinavica 73: 18–21

Phillips R A 1964 Water and electrolyte losses in cholera. Federation Proceedings 23: 705–712

Pierce N F, Banwell J G, Mitra R C, Caranos G J, Keimowitz R I, Mondal A et al 1968a Oral maintenance of water-electrolyte and acid-base balance in cholera, a preliminary report. Indian Journal of Medical Research 56: 640–645

Pierce N F, Banwell J G, Mitra R C, Caransos G J, Keimowitz R I, Mondal A et al 1968b Effect of intragastric glucose electrolyte infusion upon water and electrolyte balance in Asiatic cholera. Gastroenterology 55: 333–343

Pierce N F, Sack R B, Mitra R C, Banwell J G, Brigham K L, Fedson D S et al 1969 Replacement of water electrolyte losses in cholera by an oral glucose-electrolyte solution. Annals of Internal Medicine 70: 1173

Pizarro D, Posada G, Levine M M 1984 Hypernatraemic diarrheal dehydration treated with 'slow' (12-hour) oral rehydration therapy: A preliminary report. Journal of Pediatrics 104: 316–319

Reid E W 1902 Intestinal absorption of solutions. Journal of Physiology (London) : 28–241

Riklis E, Quastel J H 1958 Effects of cations on sugar absorption by isolated surviving guinea pig intestine. Canadian Journal of Biochemistry and Physiology 35: 347–362

Santosham M et al 1982 Oral rehydration therapy of infantile diarrheal: A controlled study of well-nourished children hospitalized in the US and Panama. New England Journal of Medicine 306(18): 1070–1076

Schedl H P, Clifton J A 1963 Solute and water absorption by the human small intestine. *Nature* (London) 199: 1264–1267

Schultz S C 1977 Sodium-coupled solute transport by small intestine: A status report. American Journal of Physiology 223: E249–254

Schultz S C, Zalunsky R 1964 Ion transport in isolated rabbit ileum: II. The interaction between active sodium and active sugar transport. Journal of General Physiology 47: 1043–1059

Sladen G F, Dawson A M 1969 Interrelationships between the absorption of glucose, sodium and water by the normal human jejunum. Clinical Science 36: 119–132

Taylor J O, Kinzie J, Hare R, Hare K 1968 Measurement of sodium flexure in human small intestine. Journal of Clinical Investigation (Abstract 0964) 27: 386

Turnberg L A, Bieberdorf F A, Morawski S G, Fordtran J S, 1970a Interrelationships of chloride, bicarbonate, sodium and hydrogen transport in the human ileum. Journal of Clinical Investigation 49: 557–567

Turnberg L A, Fordtran J S, Carter N W, Rector F C Jr 1970b Mechanisms of bicarbonate absorption and its relationship to sodium transport in the human jejunum. Journal of Clinical Investigation 49: 548–556

World Health Organization 1983 Oral rehydration therapy: an annotated bibliography, 2nd edn. Scientific Publication no 445. World Health Organization, Washington DC

Oral therapy at home for diarrhoea

In their joint statement, *The management of diarrhoea and use of oral rehydration therapy*, the World Health Organization and UNICEF recognize the vital place of therapy at home. This includes both the use of fluid containing oral rehydration salts (ORS) in properly supervized situations, and also, '. . . the use of home remedies for the early treatment of diarrhoea' which 'can be expected to result in fewer cases developing dehydration' (WHO 1983).

Therapy appropriate for severity

Diarrhoea is a disease with a wide range of severity. The most seriously ill patients may be in circulatory collapse with pH and electrolyte imbalance that requires rapid and precise correction which is so urgent that the intravenous route is indicated. Mildly ill patients only require the simplest of fluids by mouth which can, as suggested above, make a critical difference between recovery and the development of clinically apparent dehydration. The majority of cases are intermediate in severity, from mild with undetectable dehydration to moderate degrees of dehydration. In these the salt and water intake can be greatly increased by utilizing the linked sugar-sodium mechanism described in the previous section. There is some flexibility in deciding what is the appropriate rehydration intervention for the degree of severity, particularly with the milder degrees since the body's own correction mechanisms, particularly the kidneys, can restrict loss of water and salts. The range of clinical severity and appropriate rehydration interventions are shown in Table 11.1. Note that there is considerable overlap in what is appropriate rehydration.

   The advantages of early treatment by mouth are great. As the joint statement indicates, there is accumulating experience, though still rather little numerical data, which suggests that if simple rehydration is started early, the more severe degrees of dehyration and electrolyte loss do not occur. The economic benefits of earlier and simpler rehydration are also convincing. Home rehydration solutions are cheaper than ORS in most circumstances, and ORS treatment only costs one-tenth of intravenous therapy!

Table 11.1 Appropriate rehydration for clinical condition and operational circumstances

Clinical severity of diarrhoea	Appropriate rehydration
Early diarrhoea (a few loose stools)	Extra water by mouth and 'household food solutions' (e.g. rice water, carrot soup, fruit juices, weak tea)
Mild diarrhoea with no clinical dehydration apparent (but covert dehydration, loss of body weight 2–5%)	'Salt-sugar solutions' from household ingredients, possibly with extra potassium containing foods and drink
Moderate diarrhoea and dehydration (some clinical signs of dehydration and loss of body weight of 5–10%)	Glucose-electrolyte solutions (for example, ORS) possibly starch-electrolyte solutions (i.e. a more 'complete' replacement formula)
Severe diarrhoea and dehydration (loss of body weight > 10%, possibly with metabolic upset and circulatory failure)	Intravenous rehydration with Ringer's lactate, or Darrow's-dextrose or similar solutions

Note: Where the circumstances permit and there is no improvement, the rehydration method indicated in the next stage can be used. For example if diarrhoea is rather persistent but there are still no signs of clinical dehydration, instead of merely continuing with a salt-sugar solution, it is appropriate to try the more complete ORS solution if this is available.

Therapy appropriate for situation

ORS has been effectively used at a home level where there is a good supporting service of trained depot holders or community health workers. In one study it was shown to reduce the mortality rate to one-sixth of that in a control population where no home oral rehydration was available (Rahaman 1979). Often, however, ORS is reserved for use at the health centre level since 'the present annual supply of ORS packets is only enough to treat some 2 per cent of all childhood diarrhoea episodes' (WHO 1983). Consequently this section concentrates on the simpler home preparations for use in diarrhoea.

'Household food solutions' are fluids normally used and available in homes, and are suitable for the earliest stages of diarrhoea. Often these are prepared with boiling water which means they are safer for drinking. They may contain sodium, sometimes potassium and a source of glucose, such as starches, which help the absorption of salt and water in the intestines. Two examples are rice water, often found in homes in Asia, and various soups, like carrot soup, found in North African and other homes. Fruit juices, coconut water and weak teas can also be used. In every region of the world there is a need to identify available and appropriate 'household food liquids' which will be useful for home diarrhoea treatment.

'Salt and sugar solutions' are valuable in many situations because the ingredients are frequently found in ordinary kitchens, and they effectively use the glucose-sodium linked mechanism that helps to transport salt and water across the bowel wall (Clements et al 1981). Sometimes such mixtures are made from white sugar (sucrose) and cooking salt (sodium chloride). In some communities unrefined sugar or molasses is used, and this has the advantage of containing some potassium chloride and sodium bicarbonate. There may be problems of availability, measuring and acceptability of some 'salt and sugar' methods and these will be reviewed below.

Food for diarrhoea. A component of home treatment

The most dramatic aspect of diarrhoea is the acute dehydration which can be rapidly fatal, but which responds remarkably effectively to oral rehydration (OR). Less dramatic, but almost as serious is the interaction of diarrhoea and malnutrition. Home therapy has an important role against the malignant spiral of repeated diarrhoea and progressive malnutrition, but it is less well understood or accepted than oral rehydration.

In diarrhoea, children not only lose their appetites, but food is often traditionally withheld. The infection has a nutritional cost, and in some diarrhoeas the gut is damaged resulting in impaired absorption and protein leakage. Fasting does not speed recovery because in the 'rested bowel' there may be decreased digestive enzyme activity and alterations in the normal bacterial floral environment.

In undernourished children, feeding should be started once initial rehydration is complete. Even though digestion is reduced during diarrhoea there is still a significant amount of absorption. Children who were fed as much as they wanted at this stage were found to absorb about 50 per cent of the expected protein, 60 per cent of the fat and 80 per cent of the carbohydrate which was ingested (Molla et al, 1983). This is an important positive nutritional benefit. Breast feeding is particularly valuable during diarrhoea since this component of nutritional intake is little reduced (Hoyle et al, 1980). After an episode of diarrhoea, children should be given extra food for several weeks to try and ensure that they can fulfil the catch-up growth spurt and replace meagre reserves.

ENSURING THAT A GOOD TREATMENT WORKS WELL — OVERCOMING LIMITING FACTORS IN HOME THERAPY

Treatment of diarrhoea by mouth is most effective. Efficacy is not in doubt, but practical matters require careful consideration if theory is to be converted into action for those who need it. There are fundamental questions about availability, communication and acceptability.

1. Are the physical materials required for making OR solution available?
2. How can the message about oral rehydration therapy (ORT) be communicated to those who most need it?
3. What influences acceptability and use of ORT?

The situation is different in many communities, and the questions should be examined and solutions found.

Availability

Are the materials for making OR fluid available?

This includes a consideration of the ingredients for making up a rehydration fluid, the tools and methods for measuring the ingredients, and ultimately both the chemical and microbiological quality of the fluid.

The materials required for making up an OR solution include not only the salts, sugar and water, but also the instruments for measuring and containers in which to mix and store the fluid. In some programmes the main ingredients are prepacked in sachets, for example ORS, and this reduces problems concerning the availability of individual items, but there are still questions about distribution, shelf-life and those cost of such packets. In some programmes these are made available by UN agencies through the government who either manufacture, or purchase from pharmaceutical companies. In many countries government supplies are uncertain because of budgetary fluctuations and inefficiency. Some services like the pharmacies of district hospitals can make up their own packets from basic materials, particularly the sodium chloride, sodium bicarbonate, potassium chloride and glucose in the ORS formula. These are all simple compounds and should always be obtainable, but in many poor countries shortages of even essentials are common. Pharmaceutical and food manufacturing companies are bringing out commerical OR packets or fluids. The formulations are sometimes unsatisfactory, and though the quality control may be good, the price will be beyond many, and supplies will fluctuate with the pressures of the market. Careful forward planning by the programme managers can overcome many of these problems.

One organization (PATH of Canal Place, 130 Nickerson Street, Seattle, 98194, Washington, USA) has produced a large tablet which contains all the ingredients of ORS with a dispersible compound to speed up solubility in 1 litre of drinking water. Smaller tablets are also being produced commercially with a size appropriate for a cup or glassful of OR drink. A tableted form of medication is convenient because it comes in appropriate dose sizes yet is robust and suitable for bulk storage. Tablets designed to be rapidly dispersible in water are generally hygroscopic and will go soft or moist unless the atmosphere is dry. Storage in air-tight containers may be adequate protection, but if they need to be individually sealed in foil packets they may lose their economic advantage over packets of ingredients.

Simple fluid mixtures

Where specially prepared complete formula like ORS is not available, simple mixtures can be made from sugar and salt in water. These items need not be chemically pure to be physiologically effective, and will be available in most communities and usually in many homes. The use of household items makes families independent of either government official supply lines or pharmaceutical outlets, however, they are still dependent on the market availability of salt and sugar. Some of the raw products have additional benefits, for example crude sugar or molasses which contains some potassium, an important element missing from a household solution made up from refined sugar and salt. A potassium deficiency can be made up by giving children a variety of fruit or foods; mashed banana, or papaya, fresh fruit juices, lentil, soy and whole wheat flour.

The most important recent development has been the discovery that solutions in which glucose is replaced by starch, for example, rice powder, may be more effective than a sugar-based formula (see p. 155, where this is described in some detail). Some homes may not always have sugar available, but almost all will have ready access to some form of starch from the dietary staple. This means that it should be possible for most families to make their own first aid formula and to start ORT earlier. Limitations of this method are that the rice or starch powder needs to be cooked. Also, the stability of the solution is shorter than the sugar or glucose based fluids, and fermentation may start after 4–6 hours.

Water and hygiene

For any patient with diarrhoea, particularly a child who is significantly dehydrated, the first priority is to feed him with OR fluid, and its biological purity is a secondary consideration. However, if water is contaminated with faecal pathogens and used in the preparation of an OR solution, bacterial multiplication can occur, particularly at tropical temperatures. Some bacteria, for example *V. cholerae* and toxigenic *E. coli*, reproduce more rapidly than others like *Sh. flexneri*. The organisms also multiply more rapidly in a solution which contains nitrogenous material as well as ORS, compared with a fluid of pure ORS in distilled water (Black et al 1981, Shields et al 1981).

In real life situations other factors are also relevant. The bowels of children are colonized by millions of bacteria and, particularly in the tropics, some of these are potential pathogens. The water they drink and the food they eat is often contaminated with faecal organisms. In a study from The Gambia it was shown that although pathogens grew in contaminated OR fluid, there was no increase in duration or severity of disease between children treated with this solution, compared with a group given OR fluid made up with sterile water (Watkinson et al 1980). In Brazil mothers were found competent in preparing OR fluid to the correct chemical composition, but even when given sterile water, 90 per cent contaminated this with faecal coliforms when mixing the solution. Boiling the water used for OR takes time and fuel, and personal hygiene is as important as pure water.

Recommendations about rehydration should include instructions about hand washing, the use of as clean water as possible, careful storage of the

OR fluid, which should be covered and preferably kept in a refrigerator. Any of the drink which has not been used within 24 hours of mixing should be discarded.

Measuring

In order to obtain safe and effective concentrations in the OR fluids, some reliable way must be used to measure the salts and sugar. ORS packets contain the correct amounts for dissolving in 1 litre of water. Weighing ingredients is impracticable except in a pharmacy where ingredients are being prepared in bulk, and then it is essential that mixing is very thorough before packaging in small units. Volumetric measures have been recommended both for the ingredients of ORS and for sugar and salt. Morely & King (1978) suggested a set of plastic scoops of different sizes for measuring the ingredients of ORS; glucose, sodium chloride, sodium bicarbonate and potassium chloride. Mahalanabis et al (1975) noted that as 10 ml syringes were widely available in health services these could be used to measure the ingredients. Using a dry syringe and fairly fine crystalline materials, 24 ml of

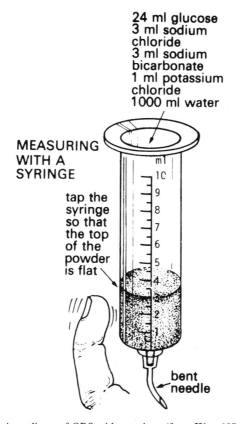

24 ml glucose
3 ml sodium chloride
3 ml sodium bicarbonate
1 ml potassium chloride
1000 ml water

MEASURING WITH A SYRINGE

tap the syringe so that the top of the powder is flat

bent needle

Fig. 11.1 Measuring ingredients of ORS with a syringe (from King 1978)

glucose, 3 ml of sodium chloride, 3 ml of sodium bicarbonate and 1 ml of potassium chloride in 1 litre of water gave a rehydration fluid with concentrations close to those of reconstituted ORS (Fig. 11.1). Locally available items can be adapted as measures. Conteh and colleagues in The Gambia (1982) found that soft drink bottle tops were widely available and could be used to measure sugar and salt. They gave sodium concentrations and osmolality results as consistent, and in a safer range than the use of teaspoons.

A plastic two-ended spoon (Hendrata 1978) has a number of attractions (see Fig. 11.2); instructions about use can be stamped onto the spoon in the local language, they are relatively cheap and reusable, facilitate the preparation of fairly consistent concentrations (Levine et al 1980), and they have a certain 'gimmick appeal'. However they also have their limitations. They are designed to measure the correct amount of sugar and salt for a particular size of cup or glass, but drinking vessels are very varied, particularly between one community and another. An additional possible source of error in mixing the correct concentration is confusing the large (sugar) and the small (salt) ends of the spoon. Another factor is the very attractiveness of the coloured plastic spoon which makes it a desirable object and plaything so that it may be stolen or lost before it is needed. Another issue is that plastic spoons depend on outside manufacture, and introduces dependence rather than encouraging the use of local products. Werner & Bower (1982, p 24.12) have shown how bottle tops and empty tin cans can be used to make two-ended sugar and salt spoons (Fig. 11.3), but without proper care, cut fingers can be a consequence of this. This is an activity for school children in a CHILD-to-child programme. A serious objection to special spoons is

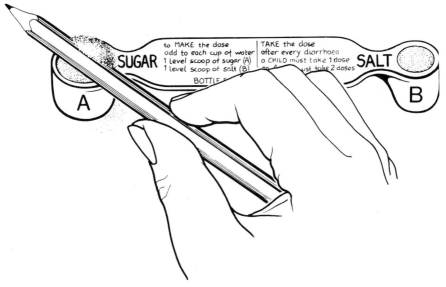

Fig. 11.2 A plastic 2-ended measuring spoon (from TALC)

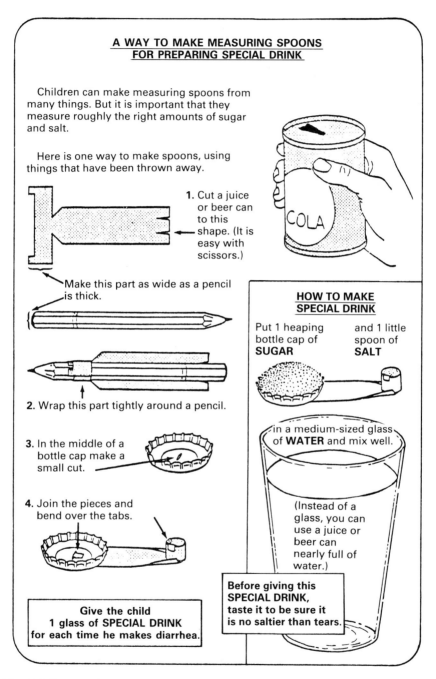

A WAY TO MAKE MEASURING SPOONS FOR PREPARING SPECIAL DRINK

Children can make measuring spoons from many things. But it is important that they measure roughly the right amounts of sugar and salt.

Here is one way to make spoons, using things that have been thrown away.

1. Cut a juice or beer can to this shape. (It is easy with scissors.)

Make this part as wide as a pencil is thick.

2. Wrap this part tightly around a pencil.

3. In the middle of a bottle cap make a small cut.

4. Join the pieces and bend over the tabs.

Give the child
1 glass of SPECIAL DRINK
for each time he makes diarrhea.

HOW TO MAKE SPECIAL DRINK

Put 1 heaping bottle cap of **SUGAR** and 1 little spoon of **SALT**

in a medium-sized glass of **WATER** and mix well.

(Instead of a glass, you can use a juice or beer can nearly full of water.)

Before giving this SPECIAL DRINK, taste it to be sure it is no saltier than tears.

Fig. 11.3 Home made measuring spoons from old cans and bottle tops (from Werner & Bower 1982)

that it depends on getting one to all families who have diarrhoea. Those who need it most urgently are from the poorest and most isolated circumstances to whom it is very difficult to distribute the spoons.

The use of the most common domestic instrument, the teaspoon, has been recommended for producing a home-made solution of suitable concentration. A 5 ml teaspoon should be filled once with salt and levelled off, and then filled and levelled 8 times with sugar (Fig. 11.4). If these 9 level teaspoonfuls are dissolved in 1 litre of drinking water the solution will contain an equivalent of 117 mmol of glucose and 85 mmol of sodium, similar amounts to the ORS which is known to be physiologically effective and safe. Although most homes have a teaspoon, their sizes are very variable and a further disadvantage is that it requires counting the number of levelled teaspoonfuls. To minimize the risk of overconcentration, if several spoon sizes and shapes are available, the recommendation is to use the smallest of the teaspoons.

For domestic rehydration using household materials it would seem appropriate to measure ingredients in the time-honoured way, using the hands of the person preparing the food or drink. This was recommended by Church (1972) (Fig. 11.5).Preliminary surveys indicated that the amount of salt picked up by a two-finger and thumb pinch was very variable (Cutting 1977). However, if a hand measuring method is taught systematically, very consistent results can be achieved (Ellerbrock 1981) (see Table 11.2).

The most important practical danger when giving OT is that a child may be given too concentrated a mixture. This can result in high blood sodium levels, hypernatraemia, that is known to have potentially harmful effects on a child's brain, possibly resulting in convulsions and haemorrhage. This could happen if a packet intended for making 1 litre (1000 ml) of fluid was made up in 200 ml. Fortunately, most children will refuse or vomit such a strong solution, but if it is forced on a passive child, without giving additional amounts of plain water, it could be harmful. There is a need for precise teaching about correct preparation. A simple practical suggestion is that before giving a child an oral rehydration mixture, the mother or whoever is administering it should taste a small amount. It should not taste too salty, definitely less salty than tears (Fig. 11.6).

There are numerous practical constraints on availability in many countries. The cash restrictions, or inappropriate use of funds by governments and families mean that there are times when money is not readily available to procure the oral rehydration fluid which can be essential and life-saving for individual patients. Even if local salt, sugar or starch is used as the basis for the therapy, there are market trends and seasonal changes that affect the availability of these. Deficient transport can be critical, whether this is due to a shortage of diesel fuel for the public transport system, or seasonal rains that put roads out of commission and make rivers impassable. These obstructions to availability can be overcome with determination, imagination and careful planning. Diarrhoea is such a common problem, and ORT such

Measuring

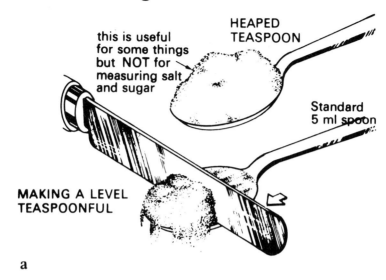

this is useful
for some things
but NOT for
measuring salt
and sugar

HEAPED
TEASPOON

Standard
5 ml spoon

MAKING A LEVEL
TEASPOONFUL

a

MAKING SALT AND SUGAR WATER

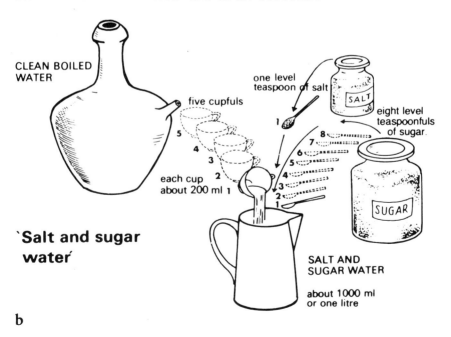

CLEAN BOILED
WATER

five cupfuls

one level
teaspoon of salt

SALT

eight level
teaspoonfuls
of sugar.

SUGAR

each cup
about 200 ml

`Salt and sugar
water´

SALT AND
SUGAR WATER

about 1000 ml
or one litre

b

Fig. 11.4 Measuring sugar and salt with a teaspoon (from King 1978)

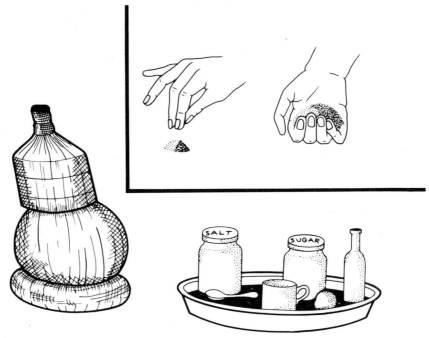

Fig. 11.5 Measuring sugar and salt by hand (after Church 1972)

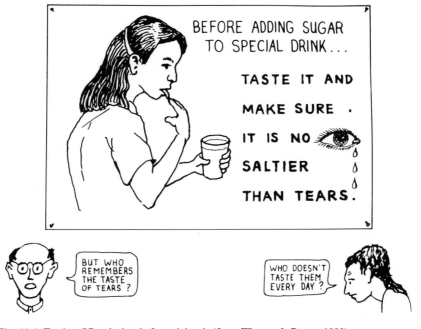

Fig. 11.6 Tasting OR solution before giving it (from Werner & Bower 1982)

an effective remedy, that ensuring supply is a worthwhile effort for a local project or a national programme.

Communication

How to get the message about ORT to those who need it?

This is not a single message, but it has a number of different component parts. The most important include:

1. Diarrhoea is a dangerous disease. (All children have diarrhoea and everyone is familiar with it, but still we must be careful as it kills many.)

2. Water and salt lost from the body is the cause of danger and death.

3. A special drink is the best treatment for diarrhoea.

4. This is how mothers can prepare and give this drink to children who need it . . . [insert here the appropriate local method for making OR fluid].

5. This really is an effective treatment. [According to the particular target audience it may be useful to give some explanation of how the treatment works].

The details of these component messages will vary according to the audience, the local materials available for preparing OR mixture and the regional policy with regard to what is the most appropriate method. There should not be too many separate messages or they cannot all be remembered. Deciding on what is the best method of OR in a community, and what should be taught is vital. This will be considered in detail below, but it is essential that the messages should be appropriate, simple and consistent (Fig. 11.7).

Groups to be reached and media for communication

The ultimate health worker is the mother, and any programme will only succeed if the parents and family 'get the message'. In many communities there will be community health workers who may be asked to help with a patient who has diarrhoea. These people are often valuable agents of change in health matters and have played a vital part in programmes that have significantly reduced the death rate from this disease (Keilmann & McCord 1977, Arole 1978). Professionals, particularly nurses and doctors, need to be well-informed and consistent on this subject or they will not provide the guidance required for such programmes. Other leaders need to know about the subject; politicians, civil servants, school teachers, religious leaders and those who set the trends in any society. Because of the varied nature of the target audience it is essential to use many methods for instruction and integrate the messages. The media for communication can conveniently be considered under three headings; publications, audio-visual and traditional. The printed word still has a great impact on many levels of society. *Diarrhoea Dialogue* is a quarterly newsletter specifically dedicated to distributing practical information about a wide variety of matters relating to the causes,

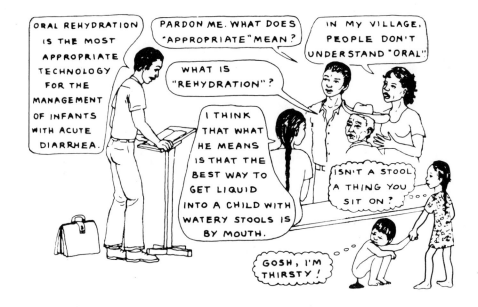

The first rule for any 'appropriate technology'
is to explain it in words that people can understand!

Fig. 11.7 Be understood — the first rule of communication (from Werner & Bower 1982)

treatment and prevention of diarrhoeal diseases. It is an independent paper, issued free of charge to all relevant workers in tropical countries, and is supported by UN and national development agencies. (*Diarrhoea Dialogue* is currently available in English, French and Spanish. An Arabic edition is planned. The address of this and other agencies distributing information on diarrhoeal disease and health education are given in Appendices 1 and 2). National and local newspapers may carry items of information about diarrhoea. These are particularly useful in reaching peripheral groups if they are in the vernacular press. In many countries picture calendars are popular. These can be imaginatively developed to convey a series of messages through pictures or cartoons. Posters are a standard form of transmitting news in some places. To be most effective these need to be carefully tested before being mass produced. Sometimes a comic-strip format may reach a significant group in a community who would never read information as prose.

Every year larger numbers of people in the world can be reached by the radiocommunication and electronic media. In some countries peasants take their transistors to work with them in the fields. Even poor countries have television networks and crowds collects around sets in front of tea shops or outside the village community centre. The cinema is still the popular entertainment medium of the Indian subcontinent and the film stars can set

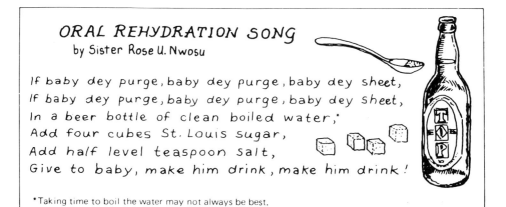

ORAL REHYDRATION SONG
by Sister Rose U. Nwosu

If baby dey purge, baby dey purge, baby dey sheet,
If baby dey purge, baby dey purge, baby dey sheet,
In a beer bottle of clean boiled water,*
Add four cubes St. Louis sugar,
Add half level teaspoon salt,
Give to baby, make him drink, make him drink!

*Taking time to boil the water may not always be best.

Fig. 11.8 A rehydration song (in Werner & Bower 1982)

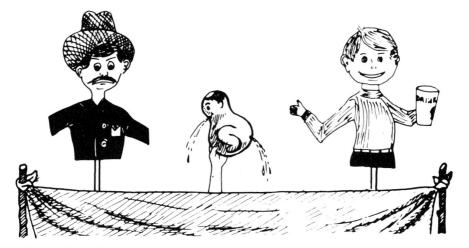

Fig. 11.9 Oral rehydration through puppet theatre (from Werner & Bower 1982)

the trend for health practices as well as other fashions. Video casettes and even the simpler slide-tape sets can be powerful tools as is demonstrated in the large supermarkets of Western countries.

The traditional ways of sharing news and entertainment should not be despised; story telling, songs and even conversation (Fig. 11.8). Professional and amateur theatre and puppet shows are always popular (Fig. 11.9, 11.10). Children in particular can be involved in a variety of play-learning activities and the CHILD-to-child programme, based at the Tropical Child Health Unit of the Institute of Child Health, has developed imaginative materials.* These and many other valuable points are made in the book

* Tropical Child Health Unit, Institute of Child Health, Guilford Street, London, WC1N 1EH, UK

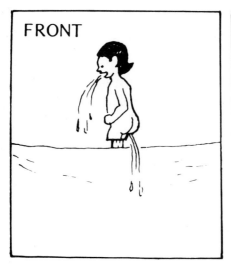
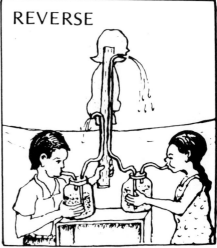

Fig. 11.10 Action puppets with the help of children (from Werner & Bower 1982)

Helping Health Workers Learn (Werner & Bower 1982) especially **15**, 10–18 and **24**, 17–29.

Integrated promotion programmes

The mass media have been effectively integrated and used in programmes in two very different countries, Honduras and The Gambia (Smith 1983). These will be described in some detail to indicate the range of communication ideas, but obviously each country needs to plan its own promotion. The impact of these programmes is now being evaluated. In Honduras the Government provides locally produced ORS called Litrosol for both home and clinic use. The radio is an important component in this context by reaching many people quickly and effectively through a large network of commercial radio stations, and many short 'spots' were used to promote oral rehydration, competing with high quality commercial advertisements. This included a 60-second song which has become a nationally popular tune. Follow-up announcements emphasize child care during diarrhoea, encouraging the administration of Litrosol and stressing the importance of continuing breast feeding during the illness. Field research in Honduras indicated that mothers associated child care with loving images. This was visually depicted by a large red heart surrounding a picture of a breast-feeding woman. This symbol was later associated with Litrosol and a young family to reinforce the role of the husband in giving ORT. The radio programmes told mothers where they could obtain Litrosol, how to mix it in the proper volume of water in containers which are readily available everywhere. (Fig. 11.11). Radio was also used to identify a network of health workers

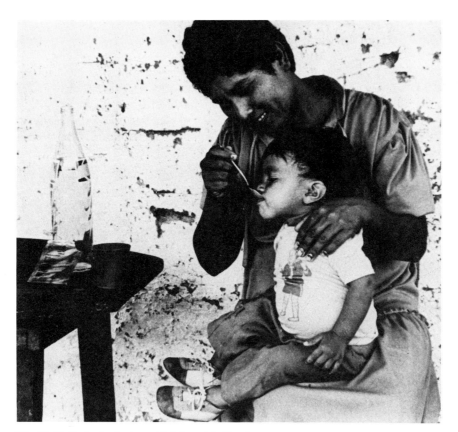

Fig. 11.11 Oral rehydration with Litrosol in Honduras

and village contacts who became known as 'red heart ladies' who had been trained to mix Litrosol. Some 1200 of these workers flew a red heart flag above their homes to attract village women to this local resource.

In the Gambia the main emphasis was to use sugar and salt at home because it was too costly to make packets available everywhere. A standard formula for the home-made solution was developed using a local soft drink (Julpearl) bottle and cap for measurements. One litre of fluid is made from three Julpearl bottles of water, 8 caps of sugar and 1 cap of salt. The correct way of preparing and giving the solution was broadcast to mothers on Radio Gambia, the national radio station. Here the information was transmitted in chatty programmes similar to others popular in the area. In addition, health questions were quickly and accurately answered in an open dialogue with mothers. The Gambian Government provided free time for hundreds of diarrhoeal-related messages on the national broadcasting system. Printed material was distributed to reinforce the message and health workers talked with mothers to make sure that they had understood. This was particularly important in the Gambia since many rural woman were unfamiliar with printed material and needed help in interpreting pictures. A colourful poster (6 in × 11 in) was developed which showed bottle and cap being used to mix the rehydration solution. The 'mixing pictures' of sugar, salt and water were colour coded and linked to explanations given over the radio. To encourage more Gambian mothers to participate in the project and to maximize the integration of radio and printed material and input by health workers, a national contest was launched popularizing the home-administered rehydration solution. Known as the 'happy baby lottery', the contest

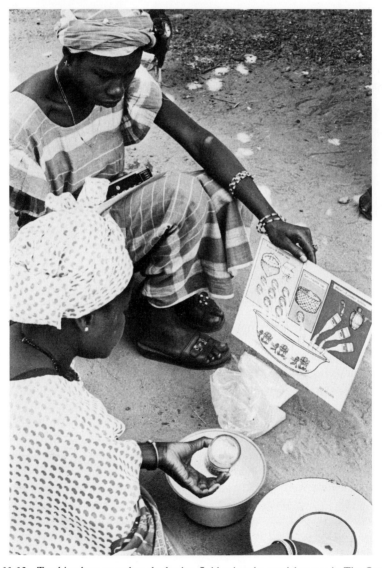

Fig. 11.12 Teaching how to make rehydration fluid using the special poster in The Gambia

helped to begin distribution of some 200 000 'mixing pictures' to mothers throughout the country. Radio Gambia broadcasted repeated programmes to rural mothers on how to use the posters as entry tickets for the context. The programmes also taught mothers how to interpret the mixing instructions on the poster. Health workers were trained how to use the posters to teach mothers how to mix the formula (Fig. 11.12). Distribution of the posters was followed by a month of 72 village contests. Every week the radio announced the names of 18 villages to be visited by a judge wearing 'happy baby' T-shirt. To enter the contest mothers went to the nearest village displaying a happy baby flag, and if they mixed the solution correctly won a prize — either a plastic litre cup or a bar of locally made soap. These prizes were chosen because they were appealing, locally available, inexpensive and consistent with the project. The response to the lottery was enthusiastic. More than 11 000 mothers attended the village contests. Over 6500 entered the mixing competition, while hundreds more watched, listened and learnt the new advice on treating diarrhoea. Winning mothers names were included in a later draw for 15 radio-cassette players. The lottery was only one part of the Gambian Government's use of mass media to fight infant diarrhoea but it stimulated tremendous interest and enthusiasm.

Acceptability

What makes people accept and use ORT?

People may know about a treatment, they may also have the materials for preparing and giving it, but what actually makes them use it?

In a recent survey in Zimbabwe (de Zoysa et al 1984) over half the people interviewed about diarrhoea knew about the treatment with a suitable fluid given by mouth, but in an area where the disease was common, only 5 per cent had actually used it in an episode of illness. The Bangladesh Rural Advancement Committee (BRAC) runs probably the biggest unipurpose oral rehydration training scheme in the world. Their trainers had covered 5 districts, 2.4 million households, nearly 15 million people by October 1983, giving individual and small group instruction and demonstrations on seven essential points of knowledge about making up and administering OR fluid. The retention of knowledge was very high, over 90 per cent of women being able to make up a safe and satisfactory rehydration mixtures even 6 months after the teaching (Table 11.2). However actual use of the solution during an episode of diarrhoea was very variable from 81 per cent to 8 per cent in different communities, with an average of 35 per cent (Chowdhury 1981). Such an important difference demands a careful review of factors influencing acceptability of the practice.

Local beliefs and practices

The application of a new idea, or the acceptance of a modified one, depends

Table 11.2   Sodium concentration in oral rehydration fluid made by village mothers from home ingredients by pinch and scoop method (from Chowdhury 1981)

Sodium conc. (mmol/l)	15 days (N = 687)	Time after teaching 3 months (N = 250)	6 months (N = 250)
Less than 30	8.9%	2.4%	0.8%
30–99	89.8%	89.6%	89.6%
100 or more	1.3%	8.0%	9.6%
Mean and s.d.	52.9 ± 20.5	65.4 ± 21.4	71.2 ± 22.0

on psychological and social factors even more than on scientific validity. With regard to diarrhoeal disease, what do people believe are the causes, and what are their traditional methods of managing the condition? These matters may not be known, even to many of the better educated people from the community itself since their beliefs will have been influenced by scientific instruction in school and college. There is a real need for simple surveys about local beliefs and practices before mounting strong promotional programmes. These should include home observation, focus group interviews and questionnaire methods. Some details about how to set about this are described in the Practical Advice section of *Diarrhoea Dialogue* 9, 6–7 (May 1982).

Some beliefs about the causes and management of diarrhoea conflict with the methods of OR, and need to be manipulated to achieve acceptance of a programme. Other beliefs obviously support the ideas of treatment by mouth. In some communities the sensible idea that dirty or unsuitable food has caused the diarrhoea leads to caution about giving anything by mouth. Similarly others believe that diarrhoea results from the failure of the bowel to absorb properly; therefore, it should be given a period of rest for recovery. The promotion of OR in such areas needs to accept these beliefs and reinterpret them as far as possible. For example, if dirty food was the cause of diarrhoea, giving significant volumes of OR fluid by mouth can be presented as a method of cleansing and washing out the poison from the system. Some believe that diarrhoea represents a 'hot' disease associated with excessive 'body heat'. For these people OR fluid can be projected as a balance of ingredients that 'cool' the system. In some countries people think that the most critical factor in severe diarrhoea is the sinking in of the soft spot or anterior fontanelle on the head of infants. They may attempt to suck this out or even raise it by pressing on the palate! Of course a sunken fontanelle is truly a danger sign in diarrhoea, but in these circumstances OT should be promoted as a vital fluid which tops up the body and literally raises the intracranial pressure along with the fluid in all the body compartments (Fig. 11.13). Traditional beliefs understood and approached in a positive way can be used to increase acceptance of ORT.

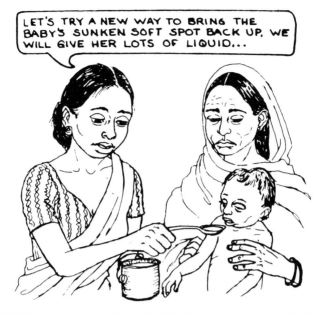

Fig. 11.13 Building on people's traditional beliefs about a sunken fontanelle (from Werner & Bower 1982)

A consistent message

Contradictory or confused instructions cannot be carried out, and a consistent message is necessary for widespread acceptability. In the survey in Zimbabwe over half the people interviewed knew that a 'special drink' was the correct treatment for diarrhoea, but when asked to make this up, most of the salt and sugar concentrations were inadequate and over 20 per cent of them were potentially dangerous. At that time there had been no recommendation about a standard method of preparing the mixture. In 1981 a literature review found 21 different methods for the preparation of a simple sugar-salt solution (Foster 1981). The calculated range of sodium level was from 8 to 289 mmol per litre (the ORS level is 90 mmol/l), and the glucose from sucrose range was 29–350 mmol per litre (ORS level 110 mmol/l). Because of such confusion it is hardly surprising that inappropriate mixtures are often prepared. If wrong mixtures are used OR will not work very well and confidence in this excellent therapy will be undermined.

The most suitable home-made or first-aid solution for a particular community will depend on basic physiological principles matched with locally available resources and traditional beliefs.

Expectations and fears

Man has long believed in the power of potions and medicines. The dramatic chemotherapeutic advances of the 20th Century have only fortified these beliefs; antibiotics can cut down bacteria in billions, anti-inflammatory drugs reduce pain and increase mobility in hours, antimitotics can seek out and destroy many malignant cells. Surely there must be a drug for diarrhoea? It comes as a disappointment, or a cause for disbelief, that the correct therapy for most cases is a simple drink. Some people demand not just treatment, but the best treatment for their child. Because intravenous infusion can have such dramatic benefits for the moribund, dehydrated patient, it may mistakenly be accepted as the optimal treatment for all cases. In point of fact, oral therapy is certainly correct and safest for cases with mild and moderate dehydration. It is unquestionably the best treatment for the majority of patients.

Oral rehydration puts the treatment of diarrhoea firmly in the hands of the family and health care aides. This clearly threatens the control of the medical professionals. Similarly, the use of home-made rehydration solutions makes people independent of pharmacies, both the commercial drug stores and the Government dispensaries. The income and control of influential groups appears threatened. Whether this factor is consciously admitted or not, it contributes to the attitude of important health professional groups to ORT.

Rehydration by mouth must not be seen as the only measure in the treatment of diarrhoea. Antibiotics are very valuable for acute dysenteric or cholera cases, and intravenous infusion can still save lives in those with severe dehydration and collapse. The danger is that man's belief in drugs and his admiration of technological intervention, displaces the essential management for the majority of cases which is quite simply drinking a suitable fluid, or ORT, to give it its scientific name.

Reinforcement of the message

To overcome reluctance to change to a new form of treatment, particularly one which may seem too simple to be credible, much positive encouragement is needed. The health services, particularly if they can speak with a unified voice, can make a big impact. The government promotional services, though sometimes regarded with suspicion, can carry a lot of weight. The leaders of other institutions in the community; school teachers, priests, monks and imams of religious organizations can add great respectability and influence any promotional programme, particularly one which centres on the welfare of many children. The role of the mass media has already been emphasized. This can be through the personal recommendation of popular personalities of the large and small screens, documentaries or through printed material of all sorts from the elegant prose of leading publications to eloquent cartoons like *Peanuts*. A mother is much more likely to try OR when her baby gets diarrhoea if she has heard about this not only from her doctor and community health worker, but is encouraged by what her older child heard at school, what father read in the newspaper, what grandmother heard on the radio and what her neighbour used for her infant last week. Drinking should become the normal response to diarrhoea.

IT REALLY WORKS!

The beauty of OR is that it really works. It provides its own evidence of effectiveness and is therefore likely to be accepted. Social science jargon for such a response may be authentication through efficacy, the personal verification of a methodology. Mothers are likely to put it more bluntly: 'That special drink saved my sister's child. Tell me what to do so I can use it for my own baby'. Until hygiene and development reduce the incidence of diarrhoea in tropical and developing countries, OR will remain a priority. Its efficacy is proven, and its simplicity means it can be used with confidence in an ordinary home (Fig. 11.14)

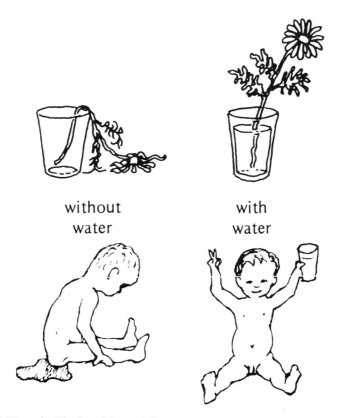

without
water

with
water

Fig. 11.14 Water for life (from Werner & Bower 1982)

APPENDIX 1

Organizations distributing information on diarrhoeal diseases

1. Diarrhoea Dialogue
   AHRTAG
   85 Marylebone High Street
   London, W1M 3DE
   UK
2. Diarrhoeal Diseases Control Programme
   World Health Organisation
   1211 Geneva 27
   Switzerland
3. International Centre for Diarrhoeal Disease Research, Bangladesh
   P.O. Box 128
   Dhaka 2
   Bangladesh
4. International Childrens Centre
   Chateau de Longchamp
   Carrefour de Longchamp
   Bois de Boulogne
   75016 Paris
   France
5. International Development Research Centre
   P.O. Box 8500
   Ottawa
   Canada, K1G 3H9
6. Ross Institute of Tropical Hygiene
   London School of Hygiene and Tropical Medicine
   Keppel Street
   London, WC1E 7HT
   UK
7. UNICEF
   Programme Development and Planning Division
   866 UN Plaza
   Room A415
   New York, NY 10017
   USA

APPENDIX 2

Sources of information on health education methods and materials

1. Academy for Educational Development
   1414 Twenty Second Street NW
   Washington DC 20037
   USA
2. British Council Media Group
   10 Spring Gardens
   London, SW1A 2BN
3. British Life Assurance Trust Centre for Health and Medical Education
   BMA House
   Tavistock Square
   London, WC1H 9JP .

4. Bureau d'Etudes et de Recherches pour la Promotion de la Sante
   B.P. 1977
   Kangu-Mayombe
   Zaire
5. Hesperian Foundation
   Box 1692
   Palo Alto, CA 94302
   USA
6. PATH
   Programme for Appropriate Technology in Health
   Canal Place
   130 Nickerson Street
   Seattle 98109
   Washington
   USA
7. PIACT de Mexico
   Shakespeare No. 27
   Mexico 5, DF
   Mexico
8. Teaching Aids at Low Cost and the
   CHILD-to-child Programme
   Tropical Child Health Unit
   30 Guilford Street
   London, WC1N 1EH, England
9. UNICEF
   Development Education Officer
   Office for Europe
   Palais des Nations
   1211 Geneva 10
   Switzerland
10. Voluntary Health Association of India
    C-14 Community Centre
    Safdarjung Development Area
    New Delhi, 100 016, India

REFERENCES

Arole R 1978 Oral rehydration therapy in the Jamkhed project. Peronsal communication
Black R E, Levine M M, Clements M L, Angle R, Robins-Brown R 1981 Proliferation of
    enteropathogens in oral rehydration solutions prepared with river water from Honduras
    and Surinam. Journal of Tropical Medicine and Hygiene 84: 195–197
Chowdhury A M R 1981 Some preliminary results from OTEP (Oral Therapy Extension
    Programme). The implications and suggested future directions. Mimeographed report
Church M A 1972 Fluids for the sick child. A method for teaching mother. Tropical Doctor
    2: 119–121
Clements M L, Levine M M, Cleaves F T, Hughes T P, Caceres M, Aleman, E et al 1981
    Comparison of simple sugar/salt versus glucose/electrolyte oral rehydration solutions in
    infant diarrhoea. Journal of Tropical Medicine and Hygiene 84: 189–194
Conteh S, McRobbie I, Tomkins A M 1982 A comparison of bottle-tops, teaspoons and
    WHO glucose-electrolyte packets for home-made oral rehydration solutions in The
    Gambia. Transactions of the Royal Society of Tropical Medicine and Hygiene
    76(6): 783–785
Cutting W A M 1977 Rehydration solutions and domestic measurements. Lancet ii: 663–4
Ellerbrock T V 1981 Oral replacement therapy in rural Bangladesh with home ingredients.
    Tropical Doctor 11: 179–183

Foster S O 1981 Household oral rehydration fluids. Personal communication

Hendrata L 1978 Spoons for making glucose-salt solution. (Correspondence) Lancet i: 612

Hoyle B, Yunus M, Chen L C 1980 Breast feeding and food intake among children with acute diarrhoeal disease. Americal Journal of Clinical Nutrition 33: 2365–2371

Kielmann A A, McCord C 1977 Home treatment of childhood diarrhoea in Punjab villages. Journal of Tropical Pediatrics and Environmental Child Health 23: 197–201

King M, King F, Martodipeoro S 1978 Primary child health. A manual for health workers. Oxford University Press, Oxford

Levine M M, Hughes T P, Black R E, Clements M L, Matheny S, Siegal A et al 1980 Variability of sodium and sucrose levels of simple sugar/salt oral rehydration solutions prepared under optimal and field conditions. Journal of Pediatrics 97(2): 324–327

Mahalanabis D, Jalan K N, Chaterjee A, Maitra T K, Agarwal S K 1975 Present and future of oral rehydration therapy for diarrhoeal diseases with special reference to health care delivery. Indian Journal of Preventive & Social Medicine 6: 286–290

Molla A, Molla A M, Sarkar S A, Khatoon N, Rahaman M M 1983 Effects of acute diarrhea on absorption of macronutrients during disease and after recovery. In: Chen L C, Scrimshaw N S (eds) Diarrhea and malnutrition, Plenum Press, New York

Morley D, King M 1978 Spoons for making glucose-salt solution. Lancet i: 53

Rahaman M M, Aziz K M S, Patwari Y, Munshi M H 1979 Diarrhoea mortality in two Bangladesh villages with and without community-based oral rehydration therapy. Lancet ii: 809–812

Shields D S, Nations-Shields M, Hook E W, Araujo J C, de Souza M A 1981 Electrolyte/glucose concentration and bacterial contamination in home-prepared oral rehydration solution: a field experience in north eastern Brazil. Journal of Pediatrics 98(5): 839–41

Smith W 1983 Delivering the goods: integrating mass media, print and visual aids. Diarrhoea Dialogue 14: 4–5

Watkinson M, Lloyd-Evans N, Watkinson A M 1980 The use of oral glucose electrolyte solution prepared with untreated well water in acute non-specific childhood diarrhoea. Transactions of the Royal Society of Tropical Medicine and Hygiene 74.5. 657–662

Werner D, Bower W 1982 Helping Health Workers Learn. Hesperian Foundation, Palo Alto, USA

World Health Organization 1983 The management of diarrhoea and use of oral rehydration therapy. A joint WHO/UNICEF statement, Geneva

de Zoysa I, Carson D, Feachem R, Kirkwood E, Lindsay-Smith E, Loewenson R 1984 Home-based oral rehydration therapy in rural Zimbabwe. Transactions of the Royal Society of Tropical Medicine and Hygiene 78: 102–105

Immunization against infectious diarrhoeas

INTRODUCTION

Diarrhoeal diseases and dysentery represent a paramount public health problem of young children in the less-developed world (Black et al 1982a, Levine & Edelman 1979, Mata 1978). The consequences of such infections include high infant mortality from diarrhoeal dehydration, malnutrition and, in some cases, chronic diarrhoea. A mere 15 years ago the aetiologic agents responsible for infant diarrhoea in the developing world were largely unrecognized; little was known about the manner in which enteropathogens evoke diarrhoea in the susceptible host; and knowledge was just beginning to accumulate concerning the secretory immune system in the intestine. At that time few less-developed countries possessed both the infrastructure and the commitment to deliver primary health care, including immunizations, to young children in rural areas and urban slums. Thus, circa 1970 it was not possible to consider immunoprophylaxis as a weapon in the battle against diarrhoeal disease. Since 1970, however, there has been a veritable explosion of knowledge concerning the aetiology of infant diarrhoea, the pathogenesis of enteric infections, and the host immune response to these agents. This new information has been applied to development of vaccines, resulting in several vaccine candidates that have reached the point of clinical trials in humans (Levine et al 1983). These developments will be discussed in this chapter.

AETIOLOGY AND EPIDEMIOLOGY OF INFANT DIARRHOEA IN RELATION TO IMMUNOPROPHYLAXIS

The epidemiology and aetiology of infant diarrhoea differ greatly between the less-developed and the industrialized countries (Levine & Edelman 1979). In less-developed countries the incidence of infant diarrhoea is very high with each child suffering an average of six to seven episodes per child per year in the first two years of life (Black et al 1982a, Levine & Edelman 1979, Mata 1978). In these areas diarrhoea manifests a peak in the warm season and bacterial diarrhoeas predominate because widespread faecal contamination of infant weaning foods, water and hands that manipulate the infant facilitate their transmission (Black et al 1982b, Levine & Edelman 1979). Among the major bacterial causes of infant diarrhoea in the less-developed countries are enterotoxigenic *Escherichia coli* (ETEC), *Campylobacter jejuni*, *Shigella*, enterpathogenic *E. coli* (EPEC) and, to a lesser extent, *Salmonella*. Approximately 60 per cent of episodes of diarrhoea in infants in less-developed areas are due to these bacterial agents, while rotavirus is considered to be the predominant viral pathogen (Black et al 1982a, Blaser et al 1983, Robins-Browne et al 1980).

At the beginning of this century similar epidemiologic patterns of infant diarrhoea existed in Europe and North America (Levine & Edelman 1979). However, over the next four decades, as industrialization and socioeconomic development proceeded accompanied by modern sanitation, enlightened hygienic practices, and widespread availability of bacteriologically monitored water and food, the incidence of infant diarrhoea plummeted and seasonality changed to a winter peak, which we now recognize to be largely due to rotavirus (Levine & Edelman 1979).

Someday all the world's population might live in conditions with modern sanitation, available potable water and improved hygiene, thereby interrupting transmission of enteropathogens to infants. However, it is unlikely that such conditions will become available in the near future to most inhabitants of rural areas and urban slums in the less-developed world, despite programmes underway to achieve these ends. In contrast, the commitment to provide primary care to such populations, including immunizations, is an achievable goal that is being ever more frequently realized in increasing numbers of less-developed countries. It is thus quite conceivable that as vaccines become available against the major causes of infant diarrhoea they could become incorporated into the routine immunization schedules for infants.

Oral rehydration with sugar/electrolytes solutions provides an important public health tool to diminish infant mortality due to diarrhoeal dehydration. However, it is important to prevent mild, non-dehydrating episodes of diarrhoea, as well as life-threatening dehydrating episodes. While, perhaps, only 1 episode of diarrhoea per 100 may result in life-threatening dehydration, all episodes of infectious diarrhoea, irrespective of aetiology, are accompanied by some degree of intestinal malabsorption which may last several weeks. Furthermore, infants consume fewer calories when ill with diarrhoea, and fever and infection per se exert a catabolic effect. For these reasons all episodes of diarrhoeal disease portend nutritional consequences which would be best averted by preventing the diarrhoeal infection itself (Black et al 1984, Mata 1978, Rosenberg et al 1977).

Village-based longitudinal studies carried out in Bangladesh suggest that effective vaccines against ETEC, rotavirus and *Shigella* could prevent approximately one-half of the episodes of diarrhoea in children in the first two years of life in that country (Black et al 1982a). As will be described below, candidate vaccines against these agents are undergoing preliminary evaluations. *C. jejuni* is becoming increasingly recognized as a pathogen in infants less than six months of life throughout the less-developed world (Blaser et al 1983), while in that same age group EPEC is important in certain geographic areas, including Brazil and South Africa (Levine & Edelman 1984). Thus, in the future, if effective vaccines were also available against *C. jejuni* and EPEC, much broader protection could be expected.

Cholera is an important cause of diarrhoeal disease in young children 2–4 years of age in endemic areas (Glass et al 1982, Mosley et al 1968). It is also a bacterial disease capable of pandemic spread and results in explosive outbreaks with high case fatality in newly affected less-developed countries. For these reasons vaccines against cholera will also be discussed.

EVIDENCE FOR INFECTION-DERIVED IMMUNITY

In considering the likelihood of success of immunoprophylaxis against infant diarrhoea, once having identified the predominant aetiologic agents, it is helpful to ascertain if evidence exists to show that prior infection with these pathogens stimulates protective immunity. As shown in Table 12.1, epidemiologic data supports the conclusion that prior natural infection with ETEC (Black et al 1981, DuPont et al 1976), *Shigella* (Levine et al 1974), rotavirus (Kapikian et al 1980) and *Vibrio cholerae* O1 (Glass et al 1982, Mosley et al 1968), confers protective immunity. Furthermore, direct evidence from experimental challenge studies in volunteers demonstrates that a prior infection with cholera (Levine et al 1981, Levine et al 1979), ETEC (Levine et al 1979b), *Shigella* (DuPont et al 1972), rotavirus (Kapikian et al 1983) or *C. jejuni* (Black et al 1983) confers significant protection against subsequent rechallenge with the homologous and sometimes strains heterologus for serotype.

ETEC and *Shigella* infections in less-developed countries exhibit a notable age-specific incidence pattern in which rates are highest in infants and young children and diminish thereafter with age (Black et al 1981). It has also been shown that the prevalence of antibody to colonization factor antigen (CFA)

Table 12.1 Evidence for infection-derived immunity in enteric infections

Pathogen	Epidemiologic studies			
	Age-specific incidence	Sero-epidemiologic	Longitudinal	Rechallenge studies in volunteers
Enterotoxigenic *E. coli*	+	+	+	+
Vibrio cholerae	+	+	+	+
Shigella	+	+	+	+
Rotavirus	+	+	+	+

+ = evidence exists

fimbriae and to heat-labile enterotoxin (LT) increases with age in children living in ETEC-endemic areas. Furthermore, the observation that adult travellers to such endemic areas from industrialized countries have high attack rates for ETEC and *Shigella* diarrhoea establishes that resistance of indigenous adults is not due to non-specific, age-related host factors but is due to specific acquired immunity.

Young adult American students newly arrived in Mexico to attend university were noted (DuPont et al 1976) to have high attack rates for ETEC diarrhoea in comparison with American students who had already lived in Mexico for at least one year and in comparison with new students from elsewhere in Latin America.

In a longitudinal study of *Shigella flexneri* 2a infections in institutionalized children (Levine et al 1974), it was noted that clinical infection occurred within the first nine months of admission to the endemic ward. Thereafter, episodic asymptomatic infections were detected for several months followed by complete absence of either clinical or subclinical infection, i.e. immunity was acquired.

By three years of age 95 per cent of young children have acquired antibodies to all rotavirus serotypes, implying that infection is almost universal in infancy and early childhood (Kapikian et al 1980). Thus rotavirus diarrhoea is uncommon beyond the third year of life. Considerable evidence also exists to show that natural cholera infection confers substantial immunity (Glass et al 1982, Mosley et al 1968).

VACCINES

Cholera vaccines

Immunizing agents against cholera will be considered first because multiple vaccine candidates have recently been evaluated. *V. cholerae* O1, the aetiologic agent of cholera, is a non-invasive bacterium that colonizes the proximal small intestine and elaborates a potent enterotoxin which results in intestinal secretion. Cholera enterotoxin (CT) consists of one biologically active A subunit and five non-toxic, immunogenic B subunits that bind the molecule to GM_1 ganglioside receptors on the enterocytes. Almost all of the neutralizing activity of antitoxin resides in antibodies to the B subunit.

For decades cholera vaccines consisted of killed whole vibrios inoculated parenterally. In field trials these vaccines provided 40–60 per cent vaccine efficacy, usually for less than 1 year (Feeley et al 1980). Protection was correlated with the titres of vibriocidal antibody induced.

Two field trials of efficacy of parenteral cholera toxoids, including glutaraldehyde cholera toxoid (Curlin et al 1975) and formaldehyde cholera toxoid (Noriki 1976), failed to give notable protection nor did glutaraldehyde cholera toxoid protect when three doses were given orally to volunteers who were subsequently experimentally challenged (Levine et al 1979a).

Recognition in recent years of the importance of the local intestinal secretory (S)IgA immune system in protection against non-invasive enteropathogens such as *V. cholerae* has stimulated interest in oral vaccines as the preferable route to maximally stimulate intestinal SIgA (Levine et al 1983). Two major avenues are being followed in developing improved cholera vaccines, one involves the use of combinations of non-living oral antigens, the other involves attenuated, non-enterotoxinogenic *V. cholerae* strains as live oral vaccines (Levine et al 1983).

Toxoid whole vibrio combination vaccines

The major attraction of non-living oral cholera vaccines is their safety. These vaccines include a toxoid component to stimulate SIgA antitoxin in combination with killed whole *V. cholerae* organisms to stimulate antibacterial immunity.

Three studies of safety and efficacy have been carried out with toxoid/whole vibrio combination vaccines (Levine et al 1983) (Table 12.2). The toxoid components have included glutaraldehyde cholera toxoid (Levine et al 1983), purified B subunit (Svennerholm et al 1982) or procholeragenoid (Finkelstein et al 1971) (the high molecular weight toxoid that results when cholera toxin is heated at 65 °C for at least 5 minutes). Each of these toxoids has been shown to be safe in humans as an oral vaccine in doses of at least 8 mg (glutaraldehyde toxoid), 5 mg (B subunit) and 200 µg (procholeragenoid).

The whole vibrio components have included alcohol-killed, heat-killed and formaldehyde-killed vibrios. Results of the three challenge studies in volunteers are shown in Table 12.2. Results were similar as all three vaccines gave moderate (27–67 per cent) vaccine efficacy and significantly diminished the severity of diarrhoea in the vaccinees. Two studies have also been carried out in volunteers immunized with oral whole vibrio vaccine without toxoid. One of these studies involved the same whole vibrio vaccine as was used in combination with B subunit; alone it gave a comparable degree of protection as was seen with the combination. These observations stress the importance of the whole cell component of the combination oral vaccines.

The disadvantages of the combination non-living antigen vaccines include the need for multiple spaced doses to prime and boost intestinal immunity, the fact that only moderate protective efficacy is induced, and the relative expense of the toxoid component (Table 12.3).

Attenuated V. cholerae *vaccines*

A prior infection in volunteers with pathogenic classical or El Tor biotype *V. cholerae* organisms induces 90–100 per cent protection against rechallenge and the immunity lasts at least three years (Levine et al 1981, Levine

Table 12.2 Comparison of efficacy of three whole vibrio/toxoid combination oral vaccines in protection against experimental cholera

Whole cell vaccine	Toxoid	No. doses	Immunization schedule (days)	Attack rate for diarrhea		Vaccine efficacy (%)	Diarrheal stool volume (ml)		Positive direct coprocultures	
				Vaccinees	Controls		Vaccinees	Controls	Vaccinees	Controls
Alcohol-killed El Tor Inaba (5×10^{10} per dose)	Glutaraldehyde-treated (2.0 mg per dose)	8 (4 doses of toxoid)	1, 4, 8, 11, 15, 19, 22, 25	2/9 $p<0.15$	4/6	67[a]	673 (585–761) $p<0.05$	1437 (834–2182)	2/9 $p<0.01$	6/6
Heat-killed classical Ogawa and Inaba; formal in-killed El Tor Inaba (10^{11} per dose)	Purified B subunit pentamer (5.0 mg per dose)	3	1, 14, 28	4/11 $p<0.01$	7/7	64[b]	700 (400–1000) $p<0.05$	3500 (300–7700)	9/11	7/7
Heat and formalin treated classical and El Tor Ogawa and Inaba (10^{11} per dose)	Procholeragenoid (50 µg for two doses, 200 µg for third dose)	3	1, 14, 28	11/15 N.S.	6/6	27[b]	1600 (300–8600) $p<0.05$	9400 (700–24 500)	14/15	6/6

[a] Challenge organism 10^6 El Tor Inaba P27459
[b] Challenge organism 10^6 El Tor Inaba N16961

Table 12.3   Comparison of new non-living antigens and live attenuated strain vaccines

	B subunit plus killed vibrio combination	Procholeragenoid plus killed whole vibrio combination	JBK 70 or CVD 101 attenuated oral vaccine strains
Number of oral doses required	3	3	1
Adverse reactions	0	0	mild diarrhoea in 20% who receive 10^6 organisms
Immunogenicity	strong antitoxin and weak antivibrio response	moderate antitoxin and weak antivibrio response	potent antivibrio response
Protective efficacy	moderate	low to moderate	high
Amelioration of illness in vaccines	yes	yes	yes

et al 1979a). This observation has led some investigators to develop attenuated strains of *V. cholerae* to serve as oral vaccines in an attempt to mimic the immunity conferred by pathogenic strains.

Naturally occurring non-enterotoxinogenic *V. cholerae* Ol strains from environmental sources in India and Brazil have been evaluated in volunteers as potential vaccine candidates with disappointing results (Levine et al 1982). These strains failed to colonize the human intestine or did so only minimally; vibriocidal antibody responses were meagre; and they did not protect in experimental challenge studies in volunteers. It thus became apparent that a live oral vaccine would have to be derived by attenuation of a pathogenic human strain.

Honda & Finkelstein (1979) mutagenized El Tor Ogawa strain 3083 with nitrosoguanidine and examined thousands of daughter colonies to detect one that continued to elaborate the immunogenic B subunit but failed to produce A subunit or holotoxin. One isolate, Texas Star-SR, fulfilled these criteria. Texas Star produces normal amounts of B subunit but is negative in assays for holotoxin activity or A subunit.

Texas Star-SR has been extensively evaluated in volunteers (Levine et al 1984b). Groups of 5 to 14 individuals were given single doses of 10^5 to 5 $\times$ 10^{10} organisms; 8 others ingested two doses of 10^9 organisms one week apart, while 18 others ingested two doses of 2 $\times$ 10^{10} organisms one week apart. Mild diarrhoea was encountered in 16 of the 68 (24 per cent) vaccinees; in only one individual did the total stool volume exceed 1.0 litre. In 35 of 46 (76 per cent) recipients of 10^8 or more vaccine organisms, the vaccine strain was cultured from duodenal fluid cultures. Hundreds of isolates recovered from clinical specimens were examined for holotoxin and found to be negative. Significant rises in serum antitoxin were detected in only 29 per cent of the vaccinees; however, 93 per cent showed significant rises in serum vibriocidal antibody.

In experimental challenge studies of vaccine efficacy in volunteers, one or two doses of Texas Star-SR were shown to confer significant protection against challenge with either El Tor Ogawa or Inaba vibrios (vaccine efficacy 61 per cent).

Although the clinical, immunological and bacteriological results of studies with Texas Star have provided important data to support the concept of using attenuated strains to mimic the immunity conferred by pathogenic *V. cholerae*, Texas Star itself suffers from certain drawbacks. These include: (i) the method of attenuation, mutagenesis with nitrosoguanidine, induces multiple point mutations, not all of which are necessarily detected, (ii) the precise genetic lesion presumably responsible for the attenuation of Texas Star is not known. Therefore, until this is elucidated there persists the theoretical possibility of reversion to virulence.

One method to overcome the possibility of reversion to toxigenicity was developed by Mekalanos et al (1982) who employed mutagenic vibriophages to delete the DNA sequences encoding cholera toxin. Deletion of DNA segments of this size eliminates the possibility to reversion and results in stable, non-enterotoxinogenic strains of *V. cholerae*. Such strains have not been tested in volunteers.

The most exciting new developments in cholera vaccines involve the preparation of non-enterotoxinogenic strains by recombinant DNA techniques (Kaper et al 1984a, 1984b, Levine et al 1984a, 1984c, Levine et al 1983, Mekalanos et al 1983). The advantages of such strains (Table 12.3) include: (i) the precise method of attenuation without compromising any other critical antigens that may be involved in immunity, (ii) complete genetic stability, and (iii) minimal expense.

An attenuated El Tor Inaba vaccine strain was prepared by Kaper et al (1984a) in which the genes encoding holotoxin were entirely deleted. This strain was fed to volunteers at doses of 10^6, 10^8 or 10^{10} viable organisms with sodium bicarbonate to neutralize the bactericidal effect of gastric acid. At the higher doses, mild diarrhoea occurred in some of the vaccinees. The vaccine strain readily colonized the proximal small intestine and stimulated a potent vibriocidal antibody response equivalent to that seen following infection with pathogenic *V. cholerae*. Most notably, a single oral dose of JBK70 vaccine conferred 89 per cent efficacy in an experimental challenge study in volunteers. This is the first vaccine ever to confer in volunteers a degree of immunity equivalent to that seen following infection with pathogenic *V. cholerae* and it accomplished this high degree of protection without stimulating cholera antitoxin (Levine et al 1984a).

Both Kaper et al (1984b) and Mekalanos et al (1983) have utilized genetic engineering techniques to prepare derivatives of classical Ogawa 395 that possess the gene encoding the B subunit but have a deletion of the gene encoding the A subunit. The strain of Kaper et al (1984b), CVD 101, was fed to volunteers in doses of 10^6, 10^7 or 10^8 organisms. Again mild diarrhoea occurred in some recipients of the higher doses. The vaccine stimulated prominent serum vibriocidal and antitoxin responses.

It is not clear why some recipients of attenuated *V. cholerae* vaccine strains such as Texas Star, JBK 70 and CVD 101, develop mild diarrhoea. It is possible that this is a consequence, per se, of colonization of the proximal small intestine by vibrios. Alternatively, it is conceivable that other entero-toxins elaborated by *V. cholerae*, distinct from cholera enterotoxin, may play a role in initiating this mild diarrhoea. Studies are underway to clarify this point. If other toxins play a role in the reactions, genes encoding these toxins can be deleted by genetic engineering an an attempt to achieve further attenuation. Clinical studies are also underway to assess the clinical ac-ceptability, intestinal colonizing capacity and immunogenicity of lower doses (10^3 to 10^5) of CVD 101 vaccine.

If the mild diarrhoea encountered in some recipients of lower doses of these genetically-engineered vaccines is simply due to the act of colonization of the proximal small intestine, this may be the price to be paid for im-munization with an inexpensive live oral vaccine that provides excellent protection after a single dose against a potentially lethal infection.

ETEC vaccines

ETEC resemble *V. cholerae* in the manner in which they cause diarrhoea. These non-invasive enteropathogens adhere to enterocytes in the proximal small intestine where they produce a heat-labile (LT) and/or a heat-stable (ST) enterotoxin. Adhesion to enterocytes is mediated by hair-like, fila-mentous, protein organelles on the surface of the ETEC called fimbriae or pili which serve as colonization factors.

Several distinct antigenic types of fimbriae that mediate attachment have been described so far in human ETEC, including colonization factor anti-gens I and II (CFA/I, CFA/II) and E8775 fimbriae. Other distinct antigenic types of colonization factor fimbriae undoubtedly exist in human ETEC pathogens and they are being sought. These fimbriae are analagous to the K88, K99 and 987-type fimbriae which exist in ETEC pathogenic for pig-lets and calves.

As with cholera, both non-living antigens and attenuated live oral vaccines are being developed (Table 12. 4).

Table 12.4 Current approaches in development of oral vaccines against enterotoxigenic *Escherichia coli*

Candidate vaccine	Immunogenic in animals	Safe	Studies in man Immunogenic	Efficacious
LT/ST toxoid	Yes	Yes	Yes	?
Purified CFA/I and II fimbriae	Yes	Yes	Minimally	No
Attenuated CFA/II-positive, non-enterotoxigenic live oral vaccine strain	Yes	Yes	Highly	Yes

Non-living ETEC vaccines

Non-living antigens, including toxoids (Furer et al 1982) and purified fimbriae (Acres et al 1979, Morgan et al 1978), have been used successfully as protective antigens in veterinary studies. In those studies pregnant sows or cows were parenterally immunized with toxoid or purified K88, K99 or 987-type fimbriae which stimulated the appearance of specific antibody in maternal milk (Acres et al 1979, Furer et al 1982, Morgan et al 1978). Newborn piglets or calves suckled on immunized mothers were significantly protected against death from diarrhoea when challenged with ETEC (bearing the homologous fimbriae), in comparison with animals suckled on non-immunized mothers. These veterinary studies have stimulated research to develop non-living purified antigens to protect against human ETEC diarrhoea. However, whereas the piglets and calves were passively protected by antibody in maternal milk, in man active immunity must be induced to achieve protection.

Klipstein et al (1983a,b) have investigated toxoids that stimulate antibody that can neutralize both LT and ST. This has been a challenge since in natural ETEC infections and experimental challenge studies in volunteers, ST (a small polypeptide) does not stimulate the appearance of neutralizing ST antitoxin. Klipstein et al (1983a,b) have chemically cross-linked biologically active synthetic ST to purified B subunit form porcine LT. (It should be noted that human and porcine LT share common antigenic determinants as well as each possessing distinct ones). The resultant toxoid retains less than 0.15 per cent of the biologically active toxigenicity of the parent LT and ST components.

The cross-linked LT/ST toxoid of Klipstein et al (1983a,b) has been tested in rats and rabbits who received either three oral doses of toxoid or a parenteral priming dose followed by oral boosters. Ligated intestinal loops were prepared in immunized and control rats and were inoculated with LT, ST and ETEC producing the toxins. The secretory response was significantly diminished in intestinal loops of immunized animals. The efficacy of this toxoid in an open gut animal model has not been reported. Klipstein et al have commenced preliminary studies with this toxoid in man (personal communication).

Other non-living antigens under evaluation as oral vaccines are purified fimbriae. Evans et al (1982) and de la Cabada et al (1981) have shown the oral immunization of rabbits with two 1.0 mg or two 5.0 mg doses of purified CFA/I fimbriae results in a significant increase in the number of anti-CFA/I-producing cells in the intestinal mucosa. When challenged enterally with an ETEC bearing CFA/I, the rabbits were protected. Preliminary studies in man with purified CFA/I have been carried out by Evans et al (personal communication).

Boedeker et al (1982) and collaborators (Levine et al 1984c) have examined purified CFA/II fimbriae as an antigen in chronic exteriorized intestinal loops of rabbits. In this model purified CFA/II stimulated prominent SIgA antifimbrial antibody responses. However, rabbits given multiple oral doses of this vaccine were not protected against enteral challenge with ETEC bearing the homologous fimbriae (M. M. Levine et al, unpublished data).

The purified CFA/II fimbriae vaccine was completely safe when fed to man but stimulated increases in SIgA intestinal and circulating IgG antiCFA/II in only 20 per cent of recipients. Not surprisingly, this vaccine, which stimulated only meagre antibody responses in only a minority of vaccines, failed to protect volunteers in an experimental challenge study (M. M. Levine et al, unpublished data).

Attenuated E. coli strains

The other approach toward prevention of ETEC diarrhoea in humans involves the use of attenuated strains bearing critical antigens as live oral vaccines (Levine 1983, Levine et al 1983). It is hoped that such strains would colonize the proximal small intestine after ingestion of a single dose and would stimulate a potent immune response to the critical antigens without causing significant untoward reactions. Recognition of critical common antigens is important since ETEC strains comprise a heterogeneous array of O:H serotypes, toxin phenotypes and fimbrial antigen types. The advent of recombinant DNA technology, however, brings into the realm of reality the construction of strains bearing multiple critical antigens of a mix never found in nature.

A prototype attenuated strain was investigated by Levine (1983) and Levine et al (1983). This strain, E1392 75–2A (provided by Dr Bernard Rowe, Colindale), is a non-enterotoxinogenic CFA/II positive variant of a previously enterotoxinogenic strain. It offered the opportunity to investigate the behaviour of an attenuated vaccine strain prototype in humans. The strain was fed to 19 volunteers in doses of 10^9, 10^{10} or 6×10^{10} organisms. Two individuals developed mild diarrhoea. The vaccine strain colonized the proximal small intestine and stimulated potent antiCFA/II responses measurable in both intestinal fluid (SIgA) and serum (IgG). The marked intestinal SIgA antiCFA/II responses after a single dose of this attenuated strain are in sharp contrast to the minimal antigenicity of multiple oral doses of purified fimbriae (Table 12.4). Based on these encouraging preliminary observations, cloned genes encoding additional critical antigens such as B subunit are being inserted into the strain by recombinant DNA techniques and the variants are being studied in man.

Shigella vaccines

In contrast to *V. cholerae* and ETEC, *Shigella* are invasive bacteria that penetrate and multiply within enterocytes of the distal small intestine and the colon. Killed parenteral vaccines consisting of whole *Shigella* organisms have proven ineffective in experimental challenge studies and in field trials. In contrast, attenuated *Shigella* strains utilized as oral vaccines have proven effective in both experimental challenge studies and field trials. The best-studied oral attenuated vaccine are the streptomycin-dependent strains of Mel et al (1971). These vaccines are not utilized in public health, however, because multiple oral doses are required to stimulate immunity and the precise genetic lesion responsible for attenuation is not known.

An exciting new development is the preparation by Formal et al (1981) of a hybrid *Shigella sonnei/Salmonella typhi* oral attenuated vaccine strain. *Salmonella typhi* Ty21a is an attenuated oral vaccine strain whose safety, genetic stability and efficacy have been confirmed in studies in volunteers as well as in field trials. Formal et al (1981) mobilized into Ty21a the 120 Mdal plasmid from *S. sonnei* that contains genes encoding production of *S. sonnei* O antigen. The resultant hybrid strain, *S. typhi* 5076–1C, produces both *S. typhi* and *S. sonnei* O antigens. This strain has been fed to volunteers and has been shown to be safe and genetically stable. Experimental challenge studies to assess vaccine efficacy are in progress.

EPEC vaccines

The classical serotype EPEC incriminated as agents of infantile diarrhoea in the 1940s and 1950s are currently recognized as a separate class of diarrhoeagenic *E. coli* that cause diarrhoea by mechanisms other than production of LT or ST or enteroinvasiveness (Levine & Edelman 1984). These *E. coli* possess a plasmid 55–65 Mdal in size that encodes genes that allow these bacteria to adhere to enterocytes resulting in a pathognomonic histopathologic lesion visible by electron microscopy (Baldini et al 1983). Investigations are underway to identify the bacterial products involved in this unique adhesion.

In the late 1960s and 1970s considerable work was carried out in Germany and Hungary with oral vaccines against EPEC including deoxycholate Boivin extract vaccines, formaldehyde-killed whole cell vaccines and attenuated streptomycin-dependent strains (Kubinyi et al 1974, Linde & Koch, 1969, Mochmann et al 1974, Rauss et al 1974). The Boivin extract vaccines were evaluated to some extent for efficacy in field trials with variable success. The streptomycin-dependent and formaldehyde-killed vaccines were not evaluated for efficacy. None of these vaccines is presently in routine use anywhere in the world.

Campylobacter jejuni vaccines

The antigenic diversity of *C. jejuni* and the pathogenesis of and immune response to infection with this agent are currently being unravelled. Thus it is too early for serious vaccine candidates and none have reached the stage of trials in man. However, it is likely that some *C. jejuni* vaccines may be available within the next few years.

Rotavirus vaccines

There is much interest in developing an effective rotavirus vaccine since this pathogen is considered to be the most important cause of viral diarrhoea in infants throughout the world. Three pieces of evidence suggest that immunization against rotavirus may be effective and is a worthy goal to pursue.

1. Orally administered gamma globulin (containing rotavirus antibody) delayed onset of excretion of rotavirus and significantly ameliorated the severity of diarrhoea in 14 rotavirus infected neonates in comparison with a control group of 11 infected neonates who received placebo (Barnes et al 1983).

2. Colostrum from cows immunized with human rotavirus and containing high titres of neutralizing antibody significantly protected Japanese orphans during a rotavirus outbreak, in comparison with controls who received milk from non-immunized cows (Ebina et al 1983).

3. A prospective study has shown that infants infected with rotavirus as neonates had significantly less frequent and less severe rotavirus infections later in infancy compared with infants who were not infected as neonates (Bishop et al 1983).

The many groups working on developing rotavirus vaccines are using several distinct approaches (Flores et al 1984, Kapikian et al 1980, Kapikian et al 1983a,b, Vesikari et al 1983, Wyatt et al 1983) (Table 12.5). These include:

Table 12.5   Strategies for development of vaccines against rotavirus

Strategy	Vaccine strains	Safety and Immunogenicity tests: Adults	Infants	Field trial of efficacy
Use of rotaviruses of animal origin	RIT 4237	+	+	+
	Bovine UK	+	−	−
	Rhesus MMU	+	+	+
Attenuation of human rotavirus by repeated passage in tissue culture	HRV5 (Wa)	+	−	−
Reassortant hybrid viruses		−	−	−
Possible natural attenuated viruses (from asymptomatic newborn nursery infections)		−	−	−
Bacteria containing rotavirus* genes encoding production of neutralization antigens				
Synthetic neutralization* antigens				

+ = test in progress
* vaccine not yet fully developed

1. Use of animal rotaviruses as possible attenuated strains.

2. Attenuating human rotaviruses by passage in tissue culture (directly or after passage in gnotobiotic animals).

3. Development of hybrid reassortant strains by coinfecting tissue cultures with both an animal strain well adapted to tissue culture and a human strain and then selecting a hybrid virus that possesses the human virus neutralization antigen but grows to high titre in tissue culture.

4. Evaluation of rotaviruses isolated from asymptomatic infected neonates in nursery outbreaks for their safety, infectivity and immunogenicity in older children on the assumption that they may be inherently attenuated.

5. Cloning a DNA copy of the RNA genes responsible for the neutralization antigen into a bacteria such as *E. coli* E1392/75–2A or attenuated *S. typhi* Ty21a. The goal is to have the bacteria express the antigen in vivo, thereby stimulating an immune response in the intestine to the rotavirus antigen (Flores et al 1984).

6. Synthetic production of the neutralization antigen and its use as a purified vaccine.

Vaccine candidates from two of the above-mentioned strategies have been tested so far in humans. Wyatt et al (1983) and Kapikian et al (1983b) fed to volunteers (having low or absent antibody titres) a human rotavirus (HRV 5 derived from Wa strain) that had been passed in gnotobiotic piglets and then in African green monkey kidney cells. Six of 10 volunteers fed this vaccine strain manifested seroconversions in rotavirus antibody but none excreted virus. Further work with this vaccine was temporarily interrupted because the virus seed was contaminated with a foamy virus. The vaccine has been repurified and further work is planned. Contamination with adventitious agents is a problem inherent in vaccine production that utilizes monkey kidney cells and underscores the desirability of cultivating vaccines in diploid cell strains.

Vesikari et al (1983) have explored the possibility of using as a vaccine in humans an animal (bovine) rotavirus that was adapted to and passed many times in tissue culture. The vaccine strain, RIT 4237, is a high passage derivative of the Nebraska Calf Diarrhoea Virus. Following a preliminary safety test in 20 healthy adults (whose rotavirus antibody levels were not reported), studies were carried out in 25 children below 2 years of age who had low or undetectable serum antibody titres to rotavirus. None of these 25 children developed gastrointestinal symptoms or other notable adverse reactions directly attributable to the vaccine. Rotavirus vaccine was not cultured from any of the children but rotaviral antigen was detectable by immunoassay in stools of 3. Seventeen of the children had no rotavirus antibody detectable by enzyme immunoassay at the time of immunization; 15 of these 17 (88 per cent) manifested significant seroconversions. Nineteen children lacked detectable neutralizing antibody pre-vaccination, but 13 of these 19 (68 per cent) seroconverted post-vaccination. Based on these encouraging preliminary studies demonstrating safety and immunogenicity in children, a successful field trial of efficacy of the RIT 4237 bovine strain was carried out in Finland (Vesikari et al 1984).

Kapikian, Wyatt and coworkers have begun studies in seronegative adult volunteers with another bovine strain from the United Kingdom which was passed many times in tissue cultures. These workers are also intending to evaluate in seronegative adult volunteers reassortant strains, a rhesus monkey strain (MMU 18006) and rotavirus strains from asymptomatic neonates. The most promising of these candidates will be further evaluated in infants.

CONCLUSION

Now that the aetiologic agents responsible for infant diarrhoea are largely identified and their virulence properties revealed, great strides have been made in developing new vaccine candidates. New vaccines against cholera, ETEC, *Shigella* and rotavirus are being evaluated in man. If some of these vaccines can be shown to be safe, effective and inexpensive, there is great confidence that they can be incorporated into primary health care immunization programmes that are increasingly reaching infants of the less-developed world. If these vaccines are successful they will diminish the occurrence of malnutrition as well as prevent deaths from diarrhoeal dehydration.

REFERENCES

Acres S D, Isaacson R E, Babiuk L A, Kapitany R A 1979 Immunization of calves against enterotoxigenic colibacillosis by vaccinating dams with purified K99 antigen and whole cell bacterins. Infection & Immunity 25: 121–126

Baldini M M, Kaper J B, Levine M M, Candy D C A, Moon H W 1983 Plasmid-mediated adhesion in enteropathogienic *Escherichia coli*. Journal of Pediatric Gastroenterology and Nutrition 2: 534–538

Barnes G L, Hewson P H, McLellan J A, Doyle L W, Knoches A M L, Kitchen W H, Bishop R F 1983 A randomized trial of oral gammaglobulin in low-birth-weight infants infected with rotavirus. Lancet ii 1371–3

Bishop R F, Barnes G L, Cirpiani E, Lund J S 1983 Clinical immunity after neonatal rotavirus infection. New England Journal of Medicine 309: 72–6

Black R E, Brown K H, Becker S 1984 Effects of diarrhea associated with specific enteropathogens on the growth of children in rural Bangladesh. Pediatrics: 73: 799–805

Black R E, Brown K H, Becker S, Alim Abdul A R M, Huq I 1982a Longitudinal studies of infectious diseases and physical growth of children in rural Bangladesh. II Incidence of diarrhoea and association with known pathogens. American Journal of Epidemiology 115: 315–324

Black R E, Brown K H, Becker S, Abdul Alim A R M, Merson M H 1982b Contamination of weaning foods and transmission of enterotoxigenic *Escherichia coli* diarrhoea in children in rural Bangladesh. Transactions of the Royal Society of Tropical Medicine and Hygiene 76: 259–64

Black R E, Levine M M, Blaser M J, Clements M L, Hughes T P 1983 Studies of *Campylobacter jejuni* infections in volutneers. In: Pearson A D, Skirrow M B, Rowe B, Davies J, Jones D M (eds) Campylobacter II. Proceedings second international workshop on *Campylobacter* infections. Public Health Laboratory Service Publication, London, p 13

Black R E, Merson M H, Rowe B, Taylor P, Abdul Alim A R M A, Gross R J, Sack D A

1981 Enterotoxigenic *Escherichia coli* diarrhoea: acquired immunity and transmission in an endemic area. Bulletin of the World Health Organization 59: 263–268

Blaser M J, Taylor D N, Feldman R A 1983 Epidemiology of *Campylobacter jejuni* infections. Epidemiologic Reviews 5: 157–76

Boedeker E C, Young C R, Collins H H, Cheney C, Levine M M 1982 Towards a vaccine for travelers' diarrhoea; mucosally-administered *E. coli* colonization factor antigens elicit a specific local immunoglobulin A response in isolated intestinal loops. Gastroenterology 82: 1020

Curlin C, Levine R, Aziz K M A, Mizanor Rahman A C M, Verway W F 1975 Field trial of cholera toxoid. In: Proceedings of the 11th joint conference on cholera. US-Japan Cooperative Medical Science Program, p 314–329

de la Cabada F J, Evans D G, Evans D J Jr 1981 Immunoprotection against enterotoxigenic *Escherichia coli* diarrhoea in rabbits by peroral administration of purified colonization factor antigen I (CFA/I). Federation of European Microbiology Societies Microbiological Letters 11: 303–307

DuPont H L, Hornick R B, Snyder M J, Libonati J P, Formal S B, Gangarosa E J 1972 Immunity in shigellosis. II Protection conferred by oral live vaccine or primary infection. Journal of Infectious Disease 125: 12–16

DuPont H L, Olarte J, Evans D G, Pickering L K, Galinda E, Evans D J 1976 Comparative susceptibility of Latin American and United States students to enteric pathogens. New England Journal of Medicine 295: 1520–1521

Ebina T, Umezu K, Ohyama S, et al. 1983 Prevention of rotavirus infection by cow colostrum containing antibody against human rotavirus. Lancet ii: 1029–30

Evans D G, de la Cabada F J, Evans D J, Jr 1982 Correlation between intestinal immune response to colonization factor antigen/I and acquired resistance to enterotoxigenic *Escherichia coli* diarrhea in an adult rabbit model. European Journal of Clinical Microbiology 1: 178–185

Feeley J C, Gangarosa E J 1980 Field trials of cholera vaccine. In: Oucherlony O, Holmgren H (eds) Cholera and related diarrhoeas. 43rd Nobel Symposium, Stockholm 1978, S Karger, Basel, p 204–210

Finkelstein R A, Fujita K, Lospallutto J J 1971 Procholeragenoid: an aggregated intermediate in the formation of choleragenoid. Journal of Immunology 107: 1043–1051

Flores J, Fereno M, Kalica A, Keith J, Kapikian A, Chanock R 1984 Molecular cloning of rotavirus genes. Implications for immunoprophylaxis. In: Chanock B, Lerner B (eds) Cold Spring Habor Symposium on modern approaches to vaccines.

Formal S B, Baron L S, Kapecko D J, Washington O, Powell C, Life C A 1981 Construction of a potential bivalent vaccine strain: introduction of *Shigella sonnei* form I antigen genes into the *galE Salmonella typhi* Ty21a typhoid vaccine strain. Infection and Immunity 34: 746–750

Furer E, Cryz S J Jr, Dorner F, Nicole J, Wanner M, Germanier R 1982 Protection against colibacillosis in neonatal piglets by immunization of dams with procholeragenoid. Infection and Immunity 35: 887–894

Glass R I, Becker S, Huq M I, Stoll B J, Kahn M U, Merson M H, Lee J V, Black R E 1982 Endemic cholera in rural Bangladesh, 1966–1980. American Journal of Epidemiology 116: 959–970

Honda T, Finkelstein R A 1979 Selection and characteristics of a *Vibrio cholerae* mutant lacking the A (ADP-ribolsylating portion of the cholera enterotoxin. Proceedings of the National Academy of Sciences of the USA 76: 2052–2056

Kaper J B, Lockman H A, Baldini M A, Levine M M 1984a Recombinant nontoxinogenic *Vibrio cholerae* strains as attenuated cholera vaccine candidates. Nature: 308: 655–658

Kaper J B, Lockman H, Baldini M M, Levine M M 1984b A recombinant live oral cholera vaccine. Biotechnology 2: 345–349

Kapikian A Z, Wyatt R G, Greeberg H B, et al. 1980 Approaches to immunization of infants and young children against gastroenteritis due to rotaviruses. Reviews of Infectious Diseases 2: 459–69

Kapikian A Z, Wyatt R G, Levine M M, Yolken R H, VanKirk D N, Dolin R, Greenberg H B, Chanock R M 1983a Oral administration of human rotavirus to volunteers: induction of illness and correlates of resistance. Journal of Infectious Diseases 147: 95–106

Kapikian A Z, Wyatt R G, Levine M M, et al. 1983b Studies in volunteers with human rotaviruses. Developments in biological standardization 53: 209–18

Klipstein F A, Engert R F, Clements J D, Houghten R A 1983a Protection against human and porcine entrotoxigenic strains of *Escherichia coli* in rats immunized with a cross-linked toxoid vaccine. Infection and Immunity 40: 924–929

Klipstein F A, Engert R F, Houghten R A 1983b Protection in rabbits immunized with a vaccine of *Escherichia coli* heat-stable toxin cross-linked to the heat-labile toxin B subunit. Infection and Immunity 40: 888–893

Kubinyi L, Kiss I, Lendvni K G 1974 Epidemiological-statistical evaluation of oral vaccination against infantile *Escherichia coli* enteritis. Acta Microbiologica Academiae Scientarium Hungaricae 21: 187–191

Levine M M 1983 Travellers' diarrhoea: prospects for successful immunoprophylaxis. Scandinavian Journal of Gastroenterology 18 (suppl 84): 121–134

Levine M M, Edelman R A 1979 Acute diarrhoeal infections in infants. I Epidemiology, treatment and immunoprophylaxis. Hospital Practice 14: 89–100

Levine M M, Edelman R 1984 Enteropathogenic *Escherichia coli* of classical serotypes associated with infant diarrhoea — epidemiology and transmission. Epidemiologic Reviews: 6: 31–51

Levine M M, Black R E, Clements M L, Cisneros L, Nalin D R, Young C R 1981 Duration of infection-derived immunity to cholera. Journal of Infectious Diseases 143: 818–820

Levine M M, Black R E, Clements M L, Cisneros L, Saah A, Nalin D R, Gill D M, Craig J P, Young C R, Ristaino P 1982 The pathogenicity of nonenterotoxigenic *Vibrio choleare* serotype Ol biotype El Tor isolated from sewage water in Brazil. Journal of Infectious Diseases 145: 296–299

Levine M M, Black R E, Clements M L, Kaper J B 1984a Present status of cholera vaccines. Biochemical Society Transactions: 12: 200–202

Levine M M, Black R E, Clements M L, Lanata C, Sears S, Honda T, Young C R, Finkelstein R A 1984b Evaluation in man of attenuated *Vibrio cholerae* El Tor Ogawa strain Texas Star-SR as a live oral vaccine. Infection and Immunity 43: 515–522

Levine M M, Black R E, Clements M L, Young C R, Boedeker E, Cheney C, Schadl P, Collins H 1984c Prevention of enterotoxigenic *Escherichia coli* diarrhoeal infection in man by vaccines that stimulate anti-adhesion (anti-pili) immunity. In: Boedeker E C (ed) Attachment of micro-organisms to the gastroentestinal mucosal surface. CRC Press, Boca Raton, Fla., pp 223–244

Levine M M, Gangarosa E J, Werner M, Morris G K 1974 Shigellosis in custodial institutions. III. Prospective clinical and bacteriologic surveillance of children vaccinated with oral attenuated shigella vaccines. Journal of Pediatrics 84: 803–806

Levine M M, Kaper J B, Black R E, Clements M L 1983 New knowledge on pathogensis of bacterial enteric infections as applied to vaccine development. Microbiological Reviews 47: 510–550

Levine M M, Nalin D R, Criag J P, Hoover D, Bergquist E J, Waterman D, Holley H P, Hornick R B, Pierce N P, Libonati J P 1979a Immunity to cholera in man: relative role of antibacterial versus antitoxic immunity. Transactions of the Royal Society of Tropical Medicine and Hygiene 73: 3–9

Levine M M, Nalin D R, Hoover D L, Bergquist E J, Hornick R B, Young C R 1979b Immunity to enterotoxigenic *Escherichia coli*. Infection and Immunity 23: 729–736

Linde K, Koch H 1969 Untersuchungen zur oralen immunisierung gegen colienteritis mit streptomycin-dependenten coli-keiman. Zentralblatt fur Bakteriologie Mikrobiologie und Hygiene. I. Abteilung Originale A — Medizinische Mikrobiologie. Infecktions Kranheiten und Parasitologie 211: 476–485

Mata L J 1978 The children of Santa Maria Cauqué: a prospective study of health and growth. The MIT Press, Cambridge, Mass

Mekalanos J J, Moseley S L, Murphy J R, Falkow S 1982 Isolation of enterotoxin structural gene deletion mutations in *Vibrio cholerae* induced by two mutagenic vibriophages. Proceedings of the National Academy of Sciences of the USA 79: 151–155

Mekalanos J J, Swartz D J, Pearson G D N, Harford N, Groyne F, de Wilde M 1983 Cholera toxin genes: nucleotide sequence, deletion analysis and vaccine development. Nature 306: 551–7

Mel D M, Gangarosa E J, Radovanovic M D 1971 Studies on vaccination against bacillary dysentery. VI. Protection of children by oral immunization with streptomycin-dependent shigella strains. Bulletin of the World Health Organization 45: 457–464

Mochmann H, Ocklitz H W, Weh L, Heinrich H 1974 Oral immunization with an extract of *Escherichia coli* enteritidis. Acta Microbiologic Academiae Scientarium Hungaricae 21: 193–196

Morgan R L, Isaacson R E, Moon H W, Brinton C C, To C C 1978 Immunization of suckling pigs against enterotoxigenic *Escherichia coli*-induced diarrheal disease by vaccination dams with purified 987 or K99 pili: protection correlates with pilus homology of vaccine and challenge. Infection and Immunity 22: 771–777

Mosley W H, Benenson A S, Barni R 1968 A serological survey for cholera antibodies in rural Each Pakistan. I. The distribution of antibody in the control population of a cholera-vaccine field-trial area and the relation of antibody titer to the pattern of endemic cholera. Bulletin of the World Health Organization 38: 327–334

Noriki H 1976 Evaluation of toxoid field trial in the Phillipines. In: Fukmi H, Zinnaka Y (eds) Proceedings of the 12th joint conference on cholera. US-Japan Cooperative Medical Science Program, Sapporo, p 302–310

Rauss K, Ketyi I, Szendrei L, Vertenyi A 1974 Immunization of infants against *Escherichia coli* enteritis. Acta Microbiologica Academiae Scientarium Hungaricae 21: 181–185

Robins-Browne R M, Still C S, Miliotis M D, et al 1980 Summer diarrhoea in African infants and children. Archives of Diseases in Childhood 55: 923–8

Rosenberg I H, Solomons N, Schneider R E 1977 Malabsorption associated with diarrhea and intestinal infections. American Journal of Clinical Nutrition 30: 1248–53

Svennerholm A-M, Sack D A, Holmgren J, Bardhan P K 1982 Intestinal antibody responses after immunization with cholera B subunit. Lancet i: 305–307

Vesikari T, Isolauri E, Delem A, D'Hondt E, Andre F E, Zissis G 1983 Immunogenicity and safety of live oral attenuated bovine rotavirus vaccine strain RIT 4237 in adults and young children. Lancet ii: 807–11

Vesikari T, Isolauri E, D'Hondt E, Delem A, Andre F E, Zissis G 1984 Protection of infants against rotavirus diarrhoea by RIT 4237 attenuated bovine rotavirus strain vaccine. Lancet i: 977–982

Wyatt R G, Kapikian A Z, Greenberg H B, Kalica A R, Flores J, Hoshino Y, Chanock R, Levine M M 1983 Development of vaccines against rotavirus disease. Progress in Food and Nutrition Science 7: 189–92

The role of water supplies and sanitation in prevention of acute diarrhoeal diseases

INTRODUCTION

Provision and proper use of water supply and excreta disposal facilities are part of the diarrhoeal diseases control strategy advocated by the Programme for the Control of Diarrhoeal Diseases at the World Health Organization. They are among the primary ways by which it is hoped that the goal of the Programme — a major reduction in diarrhoea morbidity and mortality — will be achieved. The naming of the 1980s as the International Drinking Water Supply and Sanitation Decade has underlined the expectation that these interventions will promote health. Indeed, there is a sound theoretical framework on which to base the conviction that water supplies and sanitation* facilities have a role in the prevention of diarrhoeal diseases; however, the health impact literature to support this view is surprisingly inconsistent and fraught with methodological problems (White et al 1972, Saunders & Warford 1976, Kawata 1979, Blum & Feachem 1983, Feachem et al 1983). This chapter examines first the theory and then the reported experience, drawing on a few seminal studies, on the impact of water supplies and sanitation facilities on prevention of diarrhoea, and concludes with a discussion of resource allocation to maximize impact.

POTENTIAL IMPACTS

The major aetiological agents worldwide of acute diarrhoeal diseases are transmitted primarily or exclusively by the faecal–oral route; interruption of transmission may occur by preventing human or animal faeces from entering the mouth on fingers, food, fomites or in water, or by hygienically disposing of faeces, or both. Figure 13.1 demonstrates the various ways in which transmission of diarrhoeal diseases may occur and the preventive strategies appropriate to each. Several messages emerge from this diagram. First, since transmission may occur by several pathways, reduction in overall diarrhoea morbidity may require a combination of preventive measures. Truly waterborne transmission — spread by ingestion of

---

* Sanitation is used in the narrow sense of excreta disposal in this chapter.

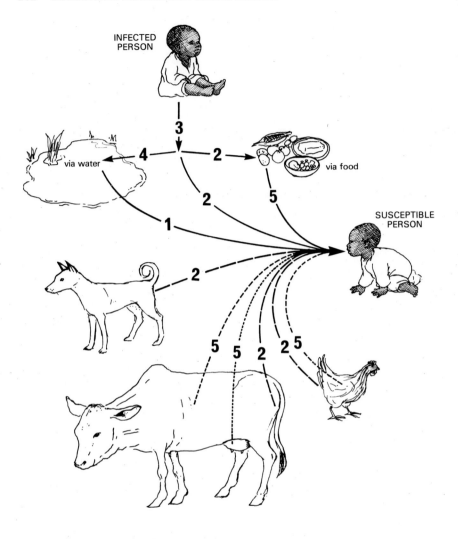

Transmission Routes

———— Human faeces

— — — Animal faeces

-------- Contaminated meat

·············· Contaminated milk

Control Measures

1 Water quality

2 Water availability plus personal and domestic cleanliness

3 Excreta disposal

4 Excreta treatment

5 Food hygiene

Fig. 13.1 The transmission and control of diarrhoeal diseases and enteric fevers. From Feachem (1983). Reproduced with the permission of The Institution of Water Engineers and Scientists, London.

an infectious agent in water — is only one of several ways by which faecal–oral spread may occur. Second, since several important transmission pathways are water-washed, that is the pathogen is passed person-to-person by a route which reflects poor personal or domestic cleanliness, interventions focused on the availability of water for hygiene may achieve greater impact than either water quality or excreta disposal interventions. While this diagram would suggest that the non-zoonotic diarrhoeal infections could be controlled simply by the provision and meticulous use by all age groups of hygienic toilets, practical considerations, especially with regard to usage of such facilities by the younger age groups, limit the usefulness of excreta disposal as the sole prevention measure. Thus it is important to try to understand the potential impacts of a variety of interventions, which may, singly or in combination, have more chance of success.

To plan appropriate preventive strategies and understand the relative merits of each, it is necessary to understand clearly the epidemiology of the important diarrhoea-causing agents in a given setting and the major factors affecting transmission: excreted load, latency (interval between excretion of an agent and its becoming infective), persistence and multiplication in the environment, infective dose, reservoirs, host immunity and host behaviour. Although there is still much to be learned about these factors for certain important agents (Feachem 1981), it is possible to classify the excreted agents, including those causing diarrhoea, according to some of these factors (Bradley 1978, Feachem et al 1983), and to formulate appropriate preventive strategies using this knowledge (Feachem 1983). Table 13.1 lists the major diarrhoea-causing agents, grouping them according to these factors, and highlights routes of transmission and the relative importance of various control strategies.

The major protozoal diarrhoeas are caused by *Entamoeba histolytica* and *Giardia lamblia* which are non-latent (immediately infective) agents, and have a low median infective dose ($<10^2$). These two factors tend to promote person-to-person spread, and may limit the impact of improvements in excreta disposal unless accompanied by changes in personal hygiene. Where there is much direct spread, the importance of waterborne transmission may be relatively limited, and hence improvements in water quality alone may achieve little measurable impact in such settings, while greater availability and use of water for personal hygiene may have much greater potential effect.

Rotavirus diarrhoea is also thought to be a non-latent, low infective dose infection but relatively little is known about its epidemiology and the factors influencing transmission. Serological surveys have shown that a high percentage of children in developed countries are infected with rotavirus by the age of 3 years (DuPont & Pickering 1980). This observation suggests that provision of adequate water supply and excreta disposal facilities are unlikely to prevent rotavirus diarrhoea worldwide. The peak incidence of ro-

Table 13.1 Transmission and control of the major diarrhoea-causing agents

Category	Agent	Major factors influencing transmission routes							Relative importance of alternative environmental control strategies[e]						
		Latency[a]	ID$_{50}$[b]	Excreted load[c]	Persistence[d]	Multiplication in the environment	Major animal reservoir	Major transmission routes	Water quality	Water availability	Excreta disposal	Excreta treatment	Personal and domestic hygiene	Drainage and sullage disposal	Food hygiene
PROTOZOA		0	L	10^5	L	No	Variable	Person-to-person contact Food Water	1	3	2	1	3	0	2
Non-latent; low infective dose	Entamoeba histolytica	0	L	10^5	L	No	No								
	Giardia lamblia	0	L	10^5	L	No	Yes								
VIRUS	(Rotavirus)	0	L (?)	10^6 (?)	H	No	No (?)	Person-to-person contact Food (?) Water (?) Air (?)	1(?)	2(?)	1(?)	1(?)	2(?)	0	1(?)

BACTERIA	Latency[a]	Median infective dose[b] (ID50)	Organisms per gram of faeces[c]	Persistence[d]	Able to multiply	Person-to-person contact[e]	Food[e]	Water[e]	Sometimes, animal-to-man contact
Non-latent; medium or high infective dose; moderately persistent; able to multiply	0	M/H	10^5–10^8	Variable	Yes	3	3	3	Variable
Campylobacter jejuni	0	M (?)	10^7	L	Yes	3	3	2	Yes
Pathogenic *E. coli*[f]	0	H	10^8	H	Yes	3	3	1	No
Salmonellae (non-typhoid)	0	H	10^8	H	Yes	3	3	1	Yes
Shigellae	0	M	10^7	M	Yes	3	1	1	No
Vibrio cholerae	0	H	10^7	M	Yes	3	2	3	No
Yersinia enterocolitica	0	H	10^5	H	Yes	3	3	1	Yes

Key
? uncertain
[a] typical minimum time from excretion to infectivity
[b] ID50 = median infective dose: L = low (<10^2) M = medium (≈10^4) H = high (>10^6)
[c] typical average number of organisms per gram of faeces
[d] estimated maximum life of infective stage at 20°–30°C: L = low (< 1 month) M = medium (≈ 1 month) H = high (> 1 month)
[e] 0 = no importance 1 = little importance 2 = moderate importance 3 = great importance
[f] includes enterotoxigenic, enteropathogenic and enteroinvasive *Escherichia coli*

Source: Adapted from Feachem (1983) and Feachem et al (1983)

tavirus diarrhoea during the colder months in temperate countries when people tend to congregate indoors suggests that person-to-person spread may be important, and hence improving water availability and personal hygiene may be appropriate preventive measures; airborne transmission remains a possibility, and if significant, will limit the usefulness of water supplies and sanitation in prevention of rotavirus diarrhoea. It is possible that prevention of rotavirus diarrhoea must await application of a vaccine.

All of the bacterial diarrhoeas are caused by agents which have a medium ($\approx 10^4$) or high ($>10^6$) median infective dose and which are non-latent and able to persist and multiply in the environment. These infections spread by waterborne and water-washed routes although the relative importance of these two routes may differ in developed and developing countries and may differ from agent to agent. Improvements in water quality and quantity are both important; excreta disposal is also important although the non-latency may promote water-washed spread even when adequate excreta disposal facilities are used.

The soil-transmitted helminths, *Trichuris trichiura* and *Strongyloides stercoralis*, are less frequent causes of diarrhoea. These helminths are latent and persistent agents with no intermediate host. Since the eggs are not immediately infective to man, personal hygiene plays a limited or negligible role in transmission. Contamination of soil is the critical factor here, and as such, sanitation control strategies are of paramount importance, particularly with *Strongyloides* which is spread exclusively by the percutaneous route.

Although the properties of the pathogens discussed above are important determinants of how faecal–oral transmission occurs, the behaviour of the human host is a critical part of the equation. The major route or routes of spread of a given diarrhoea-causing agent and the appropriate control strategy will depend both on the biology of the pathogen and the behaviour of the human host. The success of preventive measures, such as water supply and sanitation facilities, depends in turn on their maintenance and proper use. An obvious but often overlooked corollary is that it is the hygiene behaviour of those who suffer most from diarrhoeal infections and are the prime sources of infection for others that is important in determining transmission on the one hand, and success of preventive measures on the other; in many cases the group presenting the most risk are young children. Hygiene education, especially of mothers of young children, must therefore be a prime focus of any water supply and sanitation investment that hopes to have an impact on diarrhoeal diseases.

HEALTH IMPACT LITERATURE

In theory, then, water supply and sanitation, if properly maintained and used, are reasonable strategies for prevention of diarrhoea. Certainly, few would dispute the statement that poor water supply and excreta disposal have contributed to considerable diarrhoea morbidity, but how far specific improvements can be shown to lead to measurable reduction in disease or infection is by no means clear. There have been a number of recent reviews of the literature on the health impact of water supply and/or sanitation (White et al 1972, Saunders & Warford 1976, WHO 1980, McJunkin 1982, Blum & Feachem 1983, Feachem et al 1983, Hughes 1983). These reviews report over 40 studies which examine the relationship between water supply and/or sanitation and diarrhoeal disease morbidity indicators or infections related to diarrhoea. The literature is confusing and while it is tempting to derive aggregate estimates of health impact from these studies, there are great dangers in doing so. The studies are heterogeneous: in design, in the nature of environmental variables considered and in choice of impact indicators; they are often contradictory in findings; and almost all suffer from a number of methodological problems (White et al 1972, Saunders & Warford 1976, Kawata 1979, Blum & Feachem 1983, Feachem et al 1983). Interpretation of the intervention studies is hampered by a number of sampling problems and interpretation of both intervention and non-intervention studies is problematical because of one or more of the following: lack of adequate control, one-to-one comparison, confounding variables (variables such as socioeconomic status and literacy which are related both to the risk factor and outcome), health indicator recall, imprecise health indicator definition, failure to analyse by age, failure to record facility usage and failure adequately to take into account the effect of seasonality (Blum & Feachem 1983). The results of most of these studies provide little insight into how and why changes in morbidity are or are not occurring. A common combination of problems plaguing many studies includes the definition and recall of health indicators, confounding variables and failure to record facility usage.

Despite the limitations of the health impact literature as a whole, two major themes do emerge that have important implications for the environmental control of diarrhoeal diseases. First, studies that examine the impact of an environmental variable or variables on a particular diarrhoea-causing agent in the light of what is known or thought to be known about transmission of that agent, have demonstrated the importance of water availability in reducing the prevalence of *Shigella* infection (Watt et al 1953, Hollister et al 1955, Stewart et al 1955, Schliessman et al 1958) and raised questions on the efficacy of improvements in quality of drinking water in reducing the incidence of cholera or *Vibrio cholerae* infection (Sommer & Woodward 1972, Levine et al 1976, Curlin et al 1977, Spira et al 1980, Khan et al 1981, Hughes et al 1982). Second, recent studies suggest that a relatively limited water-related behavioural intervention, handwashing, can by itself, or in combination with other health and hygiene educational messages, limit the spread of acute diarrhoeal diseases and infections (Black et al 1981, Khan 1982, Torún 1982, Feachem 1984).

Many of the studies on the impact of water supply and excreta disposal on *Shigella* infection show an implicit if not always explicit recognition of the importance of person-to-person transmission and hence water availability for personal hygiene on spread of *Shigella*. In the 1950s a number of seminal studies were carried out in the United States on the isolation rates of *Shigella* in groups who differed mainly in the availability of water. Watt et al (1953) studied the prevalence of *Shigella* in children under 10 years of age in four different groups in the central San Joaquin Valley in California. As socioeconomic status, income, housing, sanitation and water availability improved, the prevalence rates decreased. In the two low socioeconomic status groups with outside water supplies, a highly significant difference in the prevalence rates of *Shigella* was found where water availability differed: the rate was 5.3 per cent in children living in homes situated close to an outdoor water tap and 9.2 per cent in children living further from a tap. Similar trends were found by Stewart et al (1955) in towns in Georgia, USA. Among otherwise similar premises, the *Shigella* infection rate was 4.1 per cent where homes were close to an outdoor water source and 5.8 per cent where the outdoor source was further away; rates were unrelated to water quality.

Hollister et al (1955), following up the earlier findings of Watt et al (1953), further investigated the influence of water availability on the prevalence of *Shigella* in children under 10 years of age in farm labour camps in the San Joaquin Valley. Children in cabins with inside water, and private shower and/or toilet had a prevalence rate of 1.6 per cent; those in cabins with inside water but with communal shower and toilet, a rate of 3.0 per cent; and those in cabins with no indoor facilities, a rate of 5.8 per cent. In those farm labour camps where all cabins used communal toilet facilities and showers but where some cabins had inside water taps and some had outside taps, the rates were 1.2 per cent among children from the former cabins and 5.9 per cent among children in the latter, although some of this difference may reflect the size of the child population in the two groups of cabins.

Schliessman et al (1958) studied the relationship of environmental factors to prevalence of *Shigella* infection among preschool children in mining camps and nearby rural hamlets in Kentucky. Among those served by outside water, no difference in *Shigella* prevalence rate was found according to proximity to the outside source, although the diarrhoea incidence rate was lower in those served by outside water located on, rather than off, the premises. The *Shigella* prevalence rate was, however, lower in the inside water-privy group (2.4 per cent) than in the outside water-privy group (5.9 per cent). The group having flush toilets and inside water had the lowest prevalence rate (1.1 per cent), suggesting that a readily available toilet offers additional benefit distinct from that of accessible water; diarrhoea morbidity was similarly affected by availability of water and/or toilets.

These studies present markedly more concordant results than the health

impact literature as a whole and, although they are not free from the methodological problems mentioned earlier, the findings are convincing in their
consistency. These studies on endemic *Shigella* infection in the United
States demonstrate a close relationship between water availability and the
prevalence of *Shigella*, with the lowest rates occurring in those with the most
plentiful supply; water quality appears unimportant in the endemic situation. There is less information on the role of excreta disposal per se on
Shigella infection, but the work of McCabe & Haines (1957) and Schliessman et al (1958) does suggest that toilets represent a useful control strategy.

It is not water availability per se which is the important factor, but rather
the amount of water used for personal hygiene. Unfortunately, none of the
Shigella studies discussed above measured the quantity of water used or
examined the relationship between infection rates and water quantity, and
none looked at water-related hygiene behaviour; all used water availability
as a substitute for quantity of water used for personal hygiene. However,
there is recent evidence from two studies in Bangladesh that water quantity
and associated human behaviour are important in prevention of shigellosis
and *Shigella* infection. Preliminary results from a large intervention programme for the control of shigellosis in Teknaf (Rahaman 1979) have shown
an inverse relationship between consumption of water (for all purposes) and
attack rates of dysentery and shigellosis. In a study in Dhaka, Bangladesh,
Khan (1982) studied a limited water-related hygiene intervention, handwashing, on transmission of *Shigella* among family members of culture-
confirmed *Shigella* patients seen at an outpatient clinic. Families were allocated
to one of four groups: a study group in which families were given water
pitchers and soap and urged to wash their hands after defaecating and before
eating; a group given only water containers; a group given only soap; and
a control group provided with neither water containers nor soap. Rectal
swabs were taken from family members daily for 10 days. The secondary
infection rate for the control group was 32.4 per cent and for the study
group 10.1 per cent, a reduction of 67 per cent. The secondary case rates
were 14.2 per cent and 2.2 per cent respectively, a reduction of 84 per cent
in the study group. Secondary infection rates were significantly lower in
those in the study group who used more water for bathing and washing; a
similar trend, although not statistically significant, was seen in the control
group. The secondary infection and case rates for the water only group were
about 32 per cent and 18 per cent respectively, and in the soap only group,
19 per cent and 5 per cent respectively, suggesting that soap is an important
factor in control. Reductions in attack rates of non-*Shigella* diarrhoea were
also found in the study group as compared to the control group, although
the difference was not statistically significant.

Two other recent studies confirm the importance of water-dependent and
other hygiene measures on spread of diarrhoea. Black et al (1981) conducted
an intervention study in 4 day-care centres in Atlanta, Georgia, and
followed diarrhoea incidence in the children for 10 months. Two of the

centres received an intensive handwashing promotion campaign and two centres received no such promotion. Diarrhoea incidence among children 6–29 months of age in the control centres was almost twice that of children in the intervention centres. In Guatemala, Torún (1982) examined the impact of health and hygiene education, as a sole intervention, on diarrhoea incidence and percentage of days ill with diarrhoea in children under 6 years of age. The educational programme emphasized not only handwashing, but also recognition and treatment of diarrhoea, excreta disposal (particularly the disposal of excreta of young children), food hygiene, care of drinking water, breast-feeding, and nutrition. During the peak diarrhoea season, there was a markedly lower incidence and proportion of days ill with diarrhoea in children in the education target group, especially in children under 2 years of age.

Whereas shigellosis may be considered a prototype water-washed disease in which person-to-person transmission is the norm in the endemic situation, cholera has classically been considered predominantly if not exclusively a waterborne disease. It follows that whereas water availability and related hygiene education is important in prevention of *Shigella* and other waterwashed infections, water quality should be important in controlling *Vibrio cholerae* and other waterborne infections. The literature on the impact of water supply and excreta disposal on cholera in developing countries is confusing as reviews on this subject by Briscoe (1978) and Feachem (1982) have pointed out. An often quoted study from the Philippines (Azurin & Alvero 1974) purports to show a marked impact of water supply and sanitation on cholera incidence. However, on closer inspection (Feachem 1982) it appears that there was no baseline data for the water intervention community and there were pre-existing differences in cholera incidence in the other communities before the interventions, making it difficult to draw definitive conclusions from the findings.

Most of the work on the influence of environmental factors, particularly water quality, on cholera incidence or *V. cholerae* infection has been done in Bangladesh and implicit in this work is the conviction that cholera is primarily waterborne. Surprisingly to those of the waterborne cholera persuasion, five studies carried out in Bangladesh (Levine et al 1976, Curlin et al 1977, Spira et al 1980, Khan et al 1981, Hughes et al 1982) have failed to show that tubewells protect against cholera or *V. cholerae* infection. A sixth study (Sommer & Woodward 1972) did find that proximity to a tubewell was associated wth a lower infection rate with the Classical biotype, but a reverse trend was found in the following year for the El Tor biotype. Briscoe (1978) explored several possible explanations for the negative findings in some of these studies, but concluded, 'We are thus left with no satisfactory explanation of the results of the tubewell studies in Matlab'.

Spira et al (1980) and Hughes et al (1982) investigated in detail transmission of *V. cholerae* among families in Matlab Thana in Bangladesh and both concluded that contaminated surface water was important in transmission. In his review of cholera epidemiology, Feachem (1982) examined each of these studies and argued that the findings are also consistent with non-waterborne transmission. The question is not so much whether or not cholera can be waterborne — waterborne cholera is well documented in the literature — but rather how much cholera is waterborne and how much is transmitted by non-waterborne faecal–oral routes. More precise knowledge of the epidemiology of *V. cholerae*, especially in the endemic situation, is needed before rational choices between alternative strategies of environmental control can be formulated. Limited intervention studies which are hypothesis-testing, such as that by Khan (1982) on the influence of handwashing on spread of *Shigella*, may be helpful in making some of these decisions. It may be that attention to personal and food hygiene may have as important a role in prevention of *V. cholerae* infection as in prevention of *Shigella* infection.

RESOURCE ALLOCATION TO MAXIMIZE IMPACT

Perhaps the most telling data on the role of water supply and excreta disposal in prevention of diarrhoeal diseases are obtained from an examination of the pattern of diarrhoea in developed countries today. In general, these countries have a reliable safe water supply and hygienic toilets which are used, and attention is paid to personal and domestic hygiene. At the same time, these countries are wealthier with higher per capita incomes, higher literacy rates and better housing than less developed countries. In this setting, there is a generally low level of endemic diarrhoeal diseases, especially among the more affluent in those countries; periodic outbreaks of diarrhoea occur, often associated with breakdowns in the water treatment process, cross-connections between potable and non-potable water or between water and sewerage systems, or deficiencies in food handling. *Vibrio cholerae, Balantidium coli, Entamoeba histolytica*, and *Salmonella typhi* are transmitted relatively infrequently. *Shigella* infection assumes a patchy distribution, occurring in crowded institutional settings, such as day-care centres, and in centres of poverty, such as farm labour camps and Indian reservations. Rotavirus is a prevalent problem, especially in children under 2 years of age during the colder months of the year. The zoonotic diarrhoeas, such as salmonellosis and campylobacteriosis, are also common. However, diarrhoea of whatever cause, when it does occur, tends to be of lesser public health importance, carrying a lower mortality, because adults and children are better nourished and able to combat infection and they have better access to medical services than is the case in developing countries.

This, then, is the situation which may evolve in many parts of the world as development proceeds and brings with it better water supply and sanitation. Morbidity and mortality due to diarrhoeal diseases should decline, although rotavirus and the zoonotic infections may remain prevalent. Water supply and sanitation, although not sufficient by themselves, are necessary interventions to achieve this improved health outlook for the future. An important question for the here and now is how to choose between various water supply, excreta disposal and hygiene control measures so as to use the often limited resources to maximize health improvements.

In theory and in practice, there is reason to believe that if much of the diarrhoea in a given setting is water-washed, a significant reduction in diarrhoea morbidity could occur with relatively limited, behaviourally orientated measures dependent on a nearby and plentiful water supply. Certainly where *Shigella* infection is common, such measures can be expected to have a significant impact. As Feachem (1981) has pointed out, it is important to understand the aetiology, epidemiology and transmission of diarrhoeal diseases in a given setting to formulate more appropriate preventive strategies. There is still much to be learned about the epidemiology and transmission of some of the major aetiologic agents worldwide of acute diarrhoeal diseases, especially *Campylobacter jejuni*, enterotoxigenic *Escherichia coli*, other enterotoxigenic bacteria, *Vibrio cholerae*, and rotavirus. Much research is needed to enable appropriate environmental and educational programmes to be established and for impacts to be meaningfully monitored. In particular, the relative importance of waterborne transmission with respect to water-washed and foodborne transmission needs to be more intensively studied using hypothesis-testing methodologies for particular agents and in various geographic settings. The pathways of transmission may well differ in developed and developing countries so that in conditions of poverty water-washed transmission assumes greater importance than waterborne transmission. In many parts of the world, low-cost technology coupled with hygiene education may prove to be a potent strategy for prevention of diarrhoeal diseases.

SUMMARY

Water supply and sanitation improvements, if properly maintained and used, are important strategies for the prevention of acute diarrhoeal diseases. All of the major diarrhoea-causing agents are transmitted by faecal-oral pathways which may be interrupted by interventions aimed at improving excreta disposal, water quality, water availability, personal and domestic hygiene, and food hygiene. The relative importance of each of these measures will depend on the epidemiology of diarrhoea in a given geographic setting and the major factors affecting transmission, including human host behaviour. The defaecation behaviour of young children is an important but often overlooked, influence on diarrhoea transmission and on the preventive potential of given interventions.

There are a number of studies which suggest that water availability and water-related hygiene behaviour (such as handwashing) are more important than water quality in prevention of acute diarrhoeal diseases in settings where there is a high likelihood of person-to-person transmission. More research is needed on the epidemiology of the major aetiologic agents of diarrhoea particularly on the relative importance of water-washed, waterborne and foodborne transmission, in order to better formulate appropriate environmental and behavioural control strategies in given settings.

ACKNOWLEDGEMENTS
The author wishes to thank David Bradley, Isabelle de Zoysa, Richard Feachem, Helen Pickering and Mujibur Rahaman for their helpful comments on earlier drafts of this chapter.

REFERENCES
Azurin J C, Alvero M 1974 Field evaluation of environmental sanitation measures against cholera. Bulletin of the World Health Organization 51: 19–26

Black R E, Dykes A C, Anderson K E et al 1981 Handwashing to prevent diarrhea in day-care centers. American Journal of Epidemiology 113: 445–451

Blum D, Feachem R G 1983 Measuring the impact of water supply and sanitation investments on diarrhoeal diseases: problems of methodology. International Journal of Epidemiology 12: 357–365

Bradley D J 1978 Towards an engineering view of health. Factors affecting the impact of sanitation on health. In: Pacey A (ed) Sanitation in developing countries. John Wiley &Sons, Chichester, ch 2, p 19–23

Briscoe J 1978 The role of water supply in improving health in poor countries (with special reference to Bangladesh). American Journal of Clinical Nutrition 31: 2100–2113

Curlin G T, Aziz K M A, Khan M R 1977 The influence of drinking tubewell water on diarrhea rates in Matlab Thana, Bangladesh. Working Paper No. 1. ICDDR, B, Dhaka, Bangladesh

DuPont H L, Pickering L K 1980 Infections of the gastrointestinal tract. Microbiology, pathophysiology, and clinical features. Plenum Medical Book Company, New York

Feachem R G 1981 Environmental and behavioural approaches to diarrheal disease control. In: Holme T, Holmgren J, Merson M H, Möllby R (eds) Acute enteric infections in children. New prospects for treatment and prevention. Elsevier/North-Holland Biomedical Press, Amsterdam, ch 15, p 289–294

Feachem R G 1982 Environmental aspects of cholera epidemiology. 111. Transmission and control. Tropical Diseases Bulletin 79: 1–47

Feachem R G 1983 Infections related to water and excreta: the health dimension of the Decade. In: Dangerfield B J (ed) Water supply and sanitation in developing countries. Water Practice Manuals, No. 3. Institution of Water Engineers and Scientists, London, ch 3, p 25–46

Feachem R G 1984 Interventions for the control of diarrhoeal diseases among young children: promotion of personal and domestic hygiene. Bulletin of the World Health Organization 62: 467–476

Feachem R G, Bradley D J, Garelick H, Mara D D 1983 Sanitation and disease. Health aspects of excreta and wastewater management. Published for the World Bank by John Wiley & Sons, Chichester

Hollister A C, Beck M D, Gittelsohn A M, Hemphill, E C 1955 Influence of water availability on Shigella prevalence in children of farm labor families. American Journal of Public Health 45: 354–362

Hughes J M 1983 Potential impacts of improved water supply and excreta disposal on diarrhoeal disease morbidity: an assessment based on a review of published studies. Unpublished Consultation Report, WHO Diarrhoeal Disease Control Programme, Geneva

Hughes J M, Boyce J M, Levine R J et al 1982 Epidemiology of El Tor cholera in rural Bangladesh: importance of surface water in transmission. Bulletin of the World Health Organization 60: 395–404

Kawata K 1979 Of typhoid fever and telephone poles: deceptive data on the effect of water supply and privies on health in tropical countries. Progress in Water Technology 11: 37–43

Khan M U 1982 Interruption of shigellosis by hand washing. Transactions of the Royal Society of Tropical Medicine and Hygiene 76: 164–168

Khan M U, Mosely W H, Chakraborty J, Sarder A M, Khan M R 1981 The relationship of cholera to water source and use in rural Bangladesh. International Journal of Epidemiology 10: 23–25

Levine R J, Khan M R, D'Souza S, Nalin D R 1976 Failure of sanitary wells to protect against cholera and other diarrhoeas in Bangladesh. Lancet: ii 86–89

McCabe L J, Haines T W 1957 Diarrhoeal disease control by improved human excreta disposal. Public Health Reports 72: 921–928

McJunkin F E 1982 Water and human health. US AID, Washington, DC

Rahaman M M 1979 A strategy for control of shigellosis (dysentery) in Teknaf — a rural Bangladesh village. Progress in Water Technology 11: 303–308

Saunders R J, Warford J J 1976 Village water supply. Economics and policy in the developing world. Johns Hopkins University Press, Baltimore

Schliessman D J, Atchley F O, Wilcomb M J, Welch S F 1958 Relation of environmental factors to the occurrence of enteric diseases in areas of eastern Kentucky. Public Health Monographs 54: 1–33

Sommer A, Woodward W E 1972 The influence of protected water supplies on the spread of Classical/Inaba and El Tor/Ogawa cholera in rural East Bengal. Lancet: ii 985–987

Spira W M, Khan M U, Saeed Y A, Sattar M A 1980 Microbiological surveillance of intra-neighbourhood El Tor cholera transmission in rural Bangladesh. Bulletin of the World Health Organization 58: 731–740

Stewart W H, McCabe L J, Hemphill E C, De Capito T 1955. IV. Diarrheal disease control studies. The relationship of certain environmental factors to the prevalence of *Shigella* infection. American Journal of Tropical Medicine and Hygiene 4: 718–724

Torún B 1982 Environmental and educational interventions against diarrhea in Guatemala. In: Chen L C, Scrimshaw N S (eds) Diarrhea and malnutrition. Interactions, mechanisms, and interventions. Plenum Press, New York, ch 15, p 235–266

Watt J, Hollister A C, Beck M D, Hemphill E C 1953 Diarrheal diseases in Fresno County, California. American Journal of Public Health 6: 728–741

White G F, Bradley D J, White A U 1972 Drawers of water. Domestic water use in East Africa. University of Chicago Press, Chicago

WHO Scientific Working Group 1980 Environmental health and diarrhoeal disease prevention. Report of a Scientific Working Group, Kuala Lumpur, Malaysia, 3–6 July 1979. WHO document DDC/80.5. World Health Organization, Geneva

The WHO diarrhoeal diseases control programme

INTRODUCTION

The acute diarrhoeal diseases have long been recognized as a major public health problem in the developing world, and since its inception, the World Health Organization has been collaborating with Member States in activities for their prevention and control.

According to a recent WHO estimate, every child under 5 years of age in the developing world suffers from, on average, 2–3 episodes of diarrhoea a year; in the first 2 years of life as many as 20 per 1000 may die from diarrhoea (Snyder & Merson 1982). This means that the acute diarrhoeal diseases cause an estimated 750–1000 million episodes of illness and some 4–5 million deaths each year in children under 5 years of age. Moreover, these repeated attacks of diarrhoea expose children to the diarrhoea–malnutrition–diarrhoea cycle, which can have long-lasting effects on the quality of life of the child. Another aspect of the problem is that diarrhoea cases in many areas of the world still account for 30 per cent or more of hospital attendances or admissions, thereby creating a heavy burden for limited national health budgets.

Until recently, these diseases were regarded as a necessary evil to be endured for decades to come until socioeconomic development reaches the level it has attained today in the industralized nations. Fortunately, however, a number of significant advances in knowledge in the past decade in the areas of diagnosis, treatment, and prevention of acute diarrhoeas have provided a solid basis for a major global attack on this vast problem. These included, among others: (i) the recognition of the role of new viral and bacterial agents as a cause of diarrhoea; (ii) a better understanding of the pathogenesis of many of the acute diarrhoeas and of the intestinal immune response, which offers new possibilities for developing better methods of treatment and prevention, including drugs and vaccines; and (iii) most important, the finding that, except in extremely severe cases, dehydration in all diarrhoeas and in all age groups can be safely and effectively treated and prevented with oral rehydration therapy (ORT).

THE WHO PROGRAMME

Recognizing the significance of these new developments, the 31st World Health Assembly in May 1978 called for a concerted attack on the diarrhoeal diseases as part of the global commitment to primary health care (PHC) and to Health for All by the Year 2000. The WHO Diarrhoeal Diseases Control (CDD) Programme was launched shortly thereafter, with the immediate objective of reducing mortality in infants and young children. Its longer term objective is to reduce the morbidity caused by diarrhoeal diseases and their associated ill effects, especially malnutrition, and to promote the self-reliance of countries in the delivery of health and social services for their control.

In order to attain its objectives, the Programme has been built up on two main components:

1. A health services (or control) component, through which WHO is actively co-operating with Member States in the development of national CDD programmes as a part of primary health care.

2. A research component, through which support is being given to health services (operational) research to determine the best ways of applying available knowledge in national control programmes, and to biomedical research to find new tools for control, especially vaccines and drugs.

Health services component

The Programme is collaborating with Member States in the development of national CDD programmes applying a package of four major control strategies (WHO 1978):

1. To reduce mortality: the *treatment* of acute diarrhoea, as early as possible in the course of illness, with ORT accompanied by the *education of mothers on appropriate feeding* of children during diarrhoea and in convalescence.

2. To reduce morbidity: the encouragement of
   a. *maternal and child care practices* that are important for the prevention of diarrhoea, especially uninterrupted breastfeeding, preparation of safe weaning foods from locally available food products and good domestic and personal hygiene
   b. *better environmental health practices*, especially the proper use and maintenance of drinking water and sanitation facilities that have been designed to conform to the needs and practices of the local population, and improved food hygiene

3. To reduce mortality and morbidity: the *detection and control of epidemics*, especially of cholera, by the establishment or strengthening of national systems for epidemiological surveillance and the introduction of measures to interrupt transmission.

The case management strategy is at present being given the highest priority, since the majority of deaths in acute diarrhoea can be prevented through ORT, comprising:

1. The *treatment* of dehydration by the use of oral rehydration salts (ORS) provided throughout the health care infrastructure;

2. The *prevention* of dehydration through promotion of the use of locally appropriate, home-prepared solutions early in the course of diarrhoea;

3. The promotion of continued proper feeding during and after diarrhoea;

4. The selective use of intravenous fluids and antibiotics.

The present joint policy of WHO and UNICEF concerning the management of diarrhoea and the use of ORT is contained in a statement published in 1983 (WHO & UNICEF 1983).

The Programme is at present undertaking an analysis of the potential impact of different interventions that could contribute to the longer-term goal of morbidity reduction, following which it should be in a position to make recommendations as to which interventions in addition to ORT can be expected to have the greatest impact on diarrhoea mortality and morbidity (Feachem et al 1983).

In the services component the Programme is collaborating with countries in incorporating existing knowledge on the treatment and prevention of diarrhoeal disease into national primary health care programmes alongside, or as an 'entry point' for other essential health care activities. WHO's activities in this respect fall into five main areas: planning of national CDD programmes, training, ORS production, communications support, and evaluation. Some of these activities can be summarized as follows:

1. As of August 1983, 65 countries had developed plans of operation for national CDD programmes and 43 of these countries had operational programmes (Table 14.1).

2. In view of the importance of proper programme management, training courses for national programme managers and for first-line supervisory staff are being organized and a planning and evaluation manual has been developed. Some 510 senior staff from 109 developing countries have already participated in the programme managers' course. Technical training for trainers is also being assured through the establishment of regional, subregional, and national training centres, and the convening of technical seminars, mostly on ORT, at the interregional, regional, and national levels. To date, 27 regional and national training centres have been established. In addition, the Programme has produced several training manuals dealing with the treatment of diarrhoea, ORS production, cholera control, and laboratory diagnosis.

3. Information on the Programme is also widely disseminated through a global newsletter *Diarrhoea Dialogue*, produced under contract by the Appropriate Health Resources and Technologies Action Group (AHRTAG) Ltd, United Kingdom, as well as through special publications such as a half-yearly *Bibliography of Acute Diarrhoeal Diseases* produced by special arrange-

Table 14.1 National CDD programmes, by region. Number of countries with plans, with operational programmes, and having conducted evaluations

Region	National CDD plan prepared[a]			National CDD programmes operational[b]	National CDD programmes evaluated[c]
	Jan. 80	April 81	July 83	July 83	July 83
Africa (AFR)	0	5	19	6	0
Americas (AMR)	2	8	13	12	3
Eastern Mediterranean (EMR)	1	2	11	8	1
Europe (EUR)	0	0	1	0	1
South-East Asia (SEAR)	5	5	9	6	1
Western Pacific (WPR)	0	4	12	11	1
Total	8	24	65	43	6

[a] A national CDD plan is one with objectives, targets, strategies, activities, budget, and a plan for evaluation. The above total comprises the following countries: *AFR*: Angola, Botswana, Benin, Burundi, Congo, Ethiopia, Gambia, Ghana, Guinea Bissau, Kenya, Mauritania, Niger, Sao Tome, Senegal, Sierra Leone, Swaziland, Togo, Uganda, Zaire; *AMR*: Belize, Bolivia, Colombia, Costa Rica, Ecuador, El Salvador, Haiti, Honduras, Jamaica, Mexico (2 states), Nicaragua, Panama, Paraguay; *EMR*: Afghanistan, Democratic Yemen, Egypt, Gaza, Jordan, Pakistan, Somalia, Sudan, Syrian Arab Republic, Tunisia, Yemen; *EUR*: Turkey; *SEAR*: Bangladesh, Bhutan, Burma, India, Indonesia, Maldives, Mongolia, Sri Lanka, Thailand; *WPR*: Fiji, Guam, Kiribati, Loas, Malaysia, Papua New Guinea, Philippines, Samoa, Solomon Islands, Tonga, Vanuatu, Viet Nam.

[b] An operational CDD programme implies the existence of a CDD unit or manager at national level, implementation of planned activities, presence of a monitoring system, and availability of ORS in at least some service facilities. The above total comprises the following countries: *AFR*: Botswana, Burundi, Congo, Ethiopia, Gambia, Sierra Leone; *AMR*: Belize, Colombia, Costa Rica, Ecuador, El Salvador, Haiti, Honduras, Jamaica, Mexico (2 states), Nicaragua, Panama, Paraguay; *EMR*: Afghanistan, Democratic Yemen, Egypt, Gaza, Jordan, Pakistan, Tunisia, Yemen; *SEAR*: Bangladesh, Burma, India, Indonesia, Sri Lanka, Thailand; *WPR*: Fiji, Kiribati, Laos, Malaysia, Papua New Guinea, Philippines, Samoa, Solomon Islands, Tonga, Vanuatu, Viet Nam.

[c] Countries conducting evaluations include: *AMR*: Ecuador, Honduras, Jamaica; *EMR*: Tunisia; *SEAR*: Thailand; *WPR*: Philippines.

ment by the National Library of Medicine, USA, and a periodic *Bibliographic Bulletin on Diarrhoeal Diseases* issued by the International Children's Centre, Paris, France (both of which are distributed by WHO in developing countries).

4. Some 30 developing countries have now taken steps to produce ORS locally, frequently with advice or support from UNICEF. Efforts are also under way to increase the stability of ORS in order to increase its shelf-life and reduce the cost of its packaging.

5. In the area of communications support, a catalogue of examples of health education materials produced by different countries has been issued and an intercountry workshop was held in one WHO region to promote the development of communication materials. Support has been given to 13 countries for the development of such materials.

6. As regards evaluation, the Programme is co-operating with governments in the undertaking of mortality and morbidity surveys to define the extent of the diarrhoeal disease problem, as well as in comprehensive programme reviews which examine the achievements and constraints of ongoing national CDD programmes. Thirty surveys and six programme reviews have

Table 14.2   Targets and projected achievements — 1989

TARGETS	
Countries with CDD programmes	100
ORS Production centres (fully operational)	24
Senior-level and front-line supervisory staff trained	2500
Subregional and national training centres	50
Country programme evaluations	80
PROJECTED ACHIEVEMENTS	
Proportion of all childhood diarrhoea cases with access to ORT	50%
Proportion of all childhood diarrhoea cases receiving ORT	37.5%
Number of childhood deaths prevented annually	1 500 000

been carried out to date.

Global targets have been set for these various activities for 1989, as well as projected achievements assuming that these targets are met (Table 14.2). A management information system has been established to monitor the progress of the Programme in achieving its objectives and to provide information for programme management at global, regional, and national levels.

Research component

The Programme's research component is regarded as an integral part of the control programme and has been designed to respond to the needs of national CDD programmes, which in turn can ensure that new research developments are rapidly applied.

An important initial step in the years 1978–1980 was the convening of nine ad hoc global Scientific Working Groups and Sub-groups, involving 64 scientists from 19 developing and 8 developed countries, to review available knowledge in a wide range of disciplines concerning diarrhoeal diseases and to determine overall research priorities for the Programme. During the same period, similar groups were convened by all six regional offices to set regional research priorities, primarily in health services (or operational) and epidemiological research. The research activities are now managed, according to the principle of peer review, by six regional and three global Scientific Working Groups. As of August 1983 the Programme had awarded support to a total of 181 (32 per cent health services and 68 per cent biomedical) research projects in 63 countries, 62 per cent of projects being in developing countries (WHO 1983a).

The Programme's research priorities in *health services research* differ somewhat from region to region and from country to country. However, certain broad priority areas are common to all regions, such as:

1. Investigations of different approaches for delivery of ORT at village and family level.

2. Aetiological studies of acute diarrhoea under different ecological and cultural conditions.

3. Studies to determine optimal ways of promoting breastfeeding and preparation of safe, locally available weaning foods.

4. Studies of traditional beliefs and practices regarding diarrhoeal diseases, and evaluation of health education approaches to modify those that are harmful.

5. Investigations of the most effective methods of environmental intervention to reduce the transmission of diarrhoeal disease agents, including methods of enlisting community participation.

In *biomedical research*, the three Scientific Working Groups are co-ordinating research in (i) bacterial enteric infections, (ii) viral diarrhoeas, and (iii) drug development and clinical management of acute diarrhoeas. The priority areas in which research is being supported are listed below:

1. Development of improved and simplified techniques for the laboratory diagnosis of the newer pathogens (e.g. rotavirus, enterotoxigenic *Escherichia coli* and *Campylobacter*);

2. Better characterization of the virulence factors in enterotoxigenic *E. coli*, *Vibrio cholerae* 01, and *Shigella;*

3. Testing and development of new vaccines against typhoid fever, cholera, rotavirus, and enterotoxigenic *E. coli*;

4. Studies on the mode of transmission of specific pathogens (especially rotavirus and *E. coli*);

5. Studies on the interrelationship of nutrition and diarrhoea (including optimal dietary therapy for children with diarrhoea);

6. Evaluation of new pharmaceutical approaches for the treatment of diarrhoea;

7. Development of alternative means of presentation of ORS.

In the important areas of vaccine and drug development, the following new approaches and developments deserve mention. A new live oral typhoid vaccine (strain Ty21a) is now being field-tested which has been shown in a first field trail in Egypt to be 96 per cent effective for three years (Wahdan et al 1982). An attempt is being made in the present trial to simplify the administration of the vaccine as an enteric coated capsule, so that it will be more suitable for general public health use. Initial plans have been made for a field trial of a new oral cholera vaccine composed of whole cells and the B-subunit of cholera toxin. Progress has also been made in the development of rotavirus vaccine: a number of candidates are at present being investigated, including a promising bovine rotavirus vaccine. Several studies are under way to develop antisecretory agents for diarrhoea and the Programme is actively collaborating with a number of pharmaceutical companies in the study of existing antidiarrhoeal drugs and compounds such as serotonin-antagonists, calcium/calmodulin inhibitors, and alpha 2 agonists.

Another important research activity initiated by the Programme is a multicentre, hospital-based, case-control study of the aetiology of diarrhoea in children under 5 years of age which is using a standard clinical and laboratory protocol to ensure the comparability of results. Multicentre studies are also under way to assess simplified tests for diagnosis of enterotoxigenic *E. coli* diarrhoea, a serotyping scheme for *C. jejuni* and an ELISA test for diagnosis of rotavirus diarrhoea.

Clinical trials are being carried out to examine the possibility of replacing sodium bicarbonate with sodium citrate to prolong the stability of ORS solution. The inclusion of amino acids and glucose polymers in the solution is also under study.

The Programme is assisted in its scientific and technical activities by a network of 11 global WHO Collaborating Centres, 3 of which have a particular responsibility for providing training for research in diarrhoeal diseases. In addition, a network of 6 developing country institutes has been established to undertake clinical drug trials.

Programme support

The Programme (WHO 1978) has aroused worldwide interest and has received the full endorsement of the Organization's Member States, as reflected in the resolution WHA35.22 adopted by the 35th World Health Assembly in May 1982 (WHO 1983b). It has benefitted from its inception from the close collaboration of UNICEF, the United Nations Development Programme (UNDP), and the World Bank, and has to date received financial support from 23 governments and agencies. The Programme budget for the biennium 1982–1983 is US $14.4 million and a total of US $20.5 million is projected for 1984–1985. However, this is only a fraction of the total that is needed to enable countries to meet the objectives of reduced mortality and morbidity due to diarrhoeal diseases, and to this effect a concerted effort will be necessary on the part of national administrators and scientists in both developing and developed countries worldwide.

REFERENCES

Feachem R, Hogan R C, Merson M H 1983 Diarrhoeal disease control: reviews of potential interventions. Bulletin of the World Health Organization 61: 637–640
Snyder J D, Merson M H 1982 The magnitude of the global problem of acute diarrhoeal disease: a review of active surveillance data. Bulletin of the World Health Organization 60: 605–613
Wahdan M H, Série C, Cerisier Y, Sallam S, Germanier P 1982 A controlled field trial of live *Salmonella typhi* strain Ty21a oral vaccine against typhoid: three-year results. The Journal of Infectious Diseases 145: 292–295
World Health Organization 1978 Control of diarrhoeal diseases: WHO's programme takes shape. WHO Chronicle 32: 369–372
World Health Organization 1983a Diarrhoeal Diseases Control Programme — Third programme report, 1981–1982. WHO Geneva (unpublished document WHO/CDD/83.8)
World Health Organization 1983b Diarrhoeal Diseases Control Programme — Progress report by the Director-General. In: Handbook of resolutions and decisions of the World Health Assembly and the Executive Board, vol II, 5th edn 1973–1982. WHO, Geneva, p 131
World Health Organization, United Nations Children's Fund 1983 The management of diarrhoea and use of oral rehydration therapy: a joint WHO/UNICEF statement. WHO, Geneva

Index